HEALING WORDS

The Power of Apology in Medicine

Second Edition

By Michael S. Woods, M.D.

Editor: Catherine Chopp Hinckley, Ph.D.
Senior Project Manager: Cheryl Firestone
Production Manager: Johanna Harris
Associate Director: Cecily Pew
Executive Director: Catherine Chopp Hinckley, Ph.D.
Vice President of Learning: Charles Macfarlane, FACHE

Cover art and book design of this edition are based on first edition work done by Polaris Creative.

Joint Commission Resources Mission

The mission of Joint Commission Resources is to continuously improve the safety and quality of care in the United States and in the international community through the provision of education and consultation services and international accreditation.

The inclusion of an organization name, product, or service in a Joint Commission Resources publication should not be construed as an endorsement of such organization, product, or services, nor is failure to include an organization name, product, or service to be construed as disapproval.

This publication is designed to provide accurate and authoritative information in regard to the subject matter covered. Every attempt has been made to ensure accuracy at the time of publication; however, please note that laws, regulations, and standards are subject to change. Please also note that some of the examples in this publication may be specific to the laws and regulations of the locality of the facility. The information and examples in this publication are provided with the understanding that neither the publisher nor the author is engaged in providing medical, legal, or other professional advice. If any such assistance is desired, the services of a competent professional person should be sought.

Requests for permission to make copies of any part of this work should be mailed to
Permissions Editor
Department of Publications
Joint Commission Resources
One Renaissance Boulevard
Oakbrook Terrace, Illinois 60181
permissions@jcrinc.com

ISBN-10: 1-59940-154-1
ISBN-13: 978-1-59940-154-6
Library of Congress Control Number: 2006934422

For more information about Joint Commission Resources, please visit http://www.jcrinc.com.

For more information about the Center for Physician Leadership, please visit http://www.doctorslead.com.

To Marcia, my closest friend, my best advisor.

To my children, who are the embodiment of love and forgiveness.

To all those brave individuals who choose to do the right thing, despite what others tell them. Stay the course.

DISCLAIMER

This material is informational only. Advice given is general. The author and publisher do not determine or assume responsibility for how or if an individual chooses to use or not use information contained herein. Providers should be familiar with their own state as well as federal laws regarding apology and disclosure, as well as the details of their liability insurance policy regarding apology and/or disclosure. They should contact their liability insurers if they have questions concerning the role of apology and/or disclosure in any situation, before speaking with any patient regarding an adverse outcome, complication, or error. Readers should consult professional counsel for specific legal, ethical, or clinical questions.

CONTENTS

Foreword vii

Introduction to the First Edition xi

Introduction to the Second Edition xiii

Chapter 1: Reclaiming Good Medicine 9

Chapter 2: A Case of Failing to Say *I'm Sorry* 13

Chapter 3: Anger in the Driver's Seat 17

Chapter 4: The Transparency Quotient 27

Chapter 5: Bedfellows and Intent: Apology and Disclosure....33

Chapter 6: Roadblocks to Apology 39

Chapter 7: Our Need for Apology 49

Chapter 8: The Five "R"s of Apology........................65

Chapter 9: Remain Engaged 77

Chapter 10: The Evidence That *I'm Sorry* Works 81

Chapter 11: The Ethical Debate About Disclosure 93

Chapter 12: Building a Culture of Civility 107

Chapter 13: Boot Camp for Authentic Relationships....115

Acknowledgments (First Edition) 127

Acknowledgments (Second Edition) 129

Resources 131

About the Author 133

Index 135

HEALING WORDS, *Second Edition*

FOREWORD
by Michael Pertschuk

As a boy, I thought that doctors were god-like, believing blindly in Michael Woods' apt, cautionary words that "modern science can perform miracles." Disillusion grew slowly, but relentlessly, as I grew older. Time and time again, I experienced or heard tales that chipped away at my faith in both the magic and the caring of doctors.

Learning to be skeptical of the limits of medicine was healthy. Learning to be skeptical of the goodness of doctors was tragic. I became increasingly convinced that too many doctors were aloof, cold, and uncaring—as arrogantly Olympian as the Greek gods, not the God of compassion. As a government official charged with consumer protection, I saw the organized medical profession lobby harder to protect physicians' income than patients' well-being. They lobbied hard to weaken or eliminate the indemnification of patients through medical malpractice law suits. But in return, they offered little self-examination. They did not recognize the failure of physicians to deal openly, honestly, and respectfully with their inevitable human errors, nor did they recognize that physicians' lack of honesty and compassion for their patients fueled patients' anger and thereby so many lawsuits.

I came to see doctors as either inherently uncaring or trained to be arrogant and cold. To me, doctors did not seem committed to caring as a calling; they seemed more concerned about the material gains from their profession than the deep satisfactions of aiding another human being in healing. And even when they *did* focus on the mechanics of healing the human body, they all too often neglected to address healing the human spirit.

What seemed to be missing most was a challenging voice—not from trial lawyers, politicians, or officious regulators like me—but a clear and passionate voice from within the profession. And then I met Mike Woods.

In the summer of 2006, I had a medical emergency—not life threatening, but something of a medical puzzle—that brought me by ambulance on July 4 to St Vincent's, our local Santa Fe hospital emergency room. Later that day, Dr. Woods came to see me and admitted me as his patient. Two days later I was discharged.

I had never been to this hospital before and knew little about it, including what to expect in the level and nature of care there. What I experienced throughout those two days, as I reflect back upon them, was an unexpected—almost startling—manifestation of the very kind of treatment that Mike Woods advocates in this vanguard book.

Happily—if only for the purposes of sampling the hospital's overall approach to patients—my ailment, ultimately diagnosed as "impressive" (Dr. Woods' bemused term), proved to be a bacterial infection, but its symptoms were atypical. As a result, Dr. Woods not only closely monitored the condition and prescribed the appropriate tests, but displayed a level of careful listening, respect, candid transparency, and an uncommon humility that I had not before encountered in the medical profession. He was also dead right in his initial diagnosis.

But he shared with me frankly his uncertainty as to the exact correctness of his diagnosis. He carefully debriefed the emergency room physician who had stayed two hours beyond her prescribed tour of duty to present her thoughts and doubts. He then called upon specialist colleagues—a cardiologist, a urologist, and an infectious disease specialist— to discuss alternative diagnoses.

The cardiologist and urologist saw nothing to dispute Dr. Woods' diagnosis. But the infectious disease specialist (after examining me carefully) stood back and with a smile, declared, "It's been very good to meet you. I have *no idea* what's wrong with you!" He then hastened to add that he thought it more likely that my symptoms indicated an allergic reaction rather than an infection (though he, again with impressive openness, said he wasn't confident enough to oppose the antibiotic treatment that Dr. Woods had ordered). He returned the next morning to say that he had researched the possibility of an allergic reaction and found some evidence that it could be a variant of hives.

Again, Dr. Woods explored openly with me this possibility, but upon subsequent examination, confirmed his original—correct—diagnosis.

Each doctor took ample time to share his or her tentative diagnosis with me, displayed patience with questions, and was gratifyingly transparent with respect to uncertainties. I must add that their not-at-all-inappropriate good humor alleviated the tension of not knowing exactly what was wrong with me.

All the doctors clearly explained to me what they knew about my condition—and more importantly, *what they didn't know.* In due course, I was well treated and cured. No mistakes marred my healing. *But if there had been a mistake, I know I would have been told fully and given an open apology. And I strongly doubt that I would ever have been moved to sue in anger and retribution.*

As Mike Woods treated me and we talked, I learned about the first edition of this book and read it with keen interest. And there I found the very description of what I had experienced: doctors who are respectful, caring, transparent, and self-reflective and who have a decidedly un-godlike readiness to have their tentative diagnosis challenged by their peers.

There is ample wise counsel in this book, some of which provides a specific antidote to medical training and acculturation, but much of which applies to all of us, health care provider and patient alike. For example, I can't help but to note how cleansing it would be to search and replace "health care provider" in this book with my own profession, "lawyer," and circulate its wise counsel to my fellow lawyers, and a few other professionals who have lost their humanity—and any trace of humility—along the way.

—Mike Pertschuk

Michael Pertschuk was the strategist in the U.S. Senate behind much of the major consumer protection and health promotion legislation of this half century; he was the most aggressive Federal Trade Commission Chair in history in pursuing health-jeopardizing marketing and promotion; and he has been a leading strategist and advocate for tobacco control for more than 40 years.

Although, by the nature of his work and role, his imprint was usually invisible, knowledgeable observers—ranging from Ralph Nader to historian Richard Kluger—have testified that no one has contributed more to the prevention of disease, injury, and death in the last half of the 20th century.

Pertschuk has had not one, but four distinct careers in public interest advocacy: (1) from 1965–1976, as consumer counsel, ultimately Chief Counsel and Staff Director to the U.S. Senate Committee on Commerce; (2) as Commissioner and Chairman of the Federal Trade Commission from 1977 to 1984; (3) from 1984 to 2004, as teacher and mentor to emerging social justice advocacy leaders and founding co-director and director of at the Advocacy Institute; and (4) as author of four books, more than 20 guides, and other writings on the art of public interest advocacy leadership.

INTRODUCTION
to the First Edition

For every medical intervention, there is an expected outcome. But there is also the possibility for unintended consequences. While it's comforting to believe modern medical science can perform miracles, the reality is that human bodies often react in unpredictable ways—even when the treatment is standardized and evidence based.

In this book, I propose that when complications occur, physicians should apologize, offer ongoing care and support, and fully disclose all details to the patient. They should never breach the patient's trust and engage in the kind of cover-ups that have become all too common in health care today. This sort of unethical behavior demeans the practice of medicine and fosters a mindset that interferes with our ability to act effectively as healers.

I believe—and statistics support this—that, when dealt with honestly, respectfully, and compassionately, patients will accept an apology and choose not to litigate. Instead, they will accept a fair financial remedy that covers the costs of additional care made necessary by the complication.

What I'm proposing in this book is simple, but profoundly important. I'm encouraging my fellow physicians to practice a common courtesy played out on the street every day. Just as a stranger automatically apologizes for unintentionally bumping into someone on a sidewalk, an apology should be the norm if a doctor is running late, interrupts a patient to take a phone call, misplaces a file—or initiates care that results in an unexpected or life-threatening outcome.

I believe most physicians long to do the right thing. When one of our patients is in pain, suffers an unanticipated outcome, or fails to respond to treatment, our hearts tell us to empathize, to reach out. Unfortunately, our profession has become increasingly deaf to the calls of the heart. Only we can change this situation.

A word of caution is in order. I believe that saying *I'm sorry* is the right thing to do, and this book contains accurate information on the value of apology in doctor-patient relationships as well as its ability to reduce malpractice claims. Despite this, some malpractice policies are written in such a way that physicians risk loss of coverage by offering an apology or information to a patient without getting prior clearance from the insurer. You must understand what your policy states concerning this issue before following my advice.

Finally, if this book fails to meet the expectations of the reader, I would like to say *I'm sorry* in advance.

INTRODUCTION
to the Second Edition

When *Healing Words* was published in early 2004, after nearly three years in the making, I thought it was an important contribution to the discussion regarding solutions to the medical malpractice debate. Little did I know the book would be on the front end of a tsunami of interest on the subject of apology and disclosure. It seemed that within months of its publication, one couldn't pick up a newspaper without seeing an article on the topic.

Unquestionably, the first edition of *Healing Words* benefited from the noise level around apology in health care. We printed 2,500 copies on the first run. It wasn't long after that until we printed another 2,500. And then 10,000 more. *Healing Words* sold 5,000 copies in just 18 months, which, remarkably, is realized by only 2% of published books, according to Nielsen BookScan. The book has been translated into Spanish for the Latin American markets of Argentina and Brazil. I speak to audiences ranging from 5 to 1,500 on the topic . . . one that I am passionate about. All of this is a result of the importance of the topic and the material itself, for I remain an imperfect messenger bearing a good and worthy message: Doing the right thing is, well, the right thing.

Despite what can only be described as a successful and well-received book, I am not satisfied with the way things stand. Sometimes success is not enough. After multiple trips and presentations, debates, discussions, and more personal experiences as a practicing surgeon, I have learned more. I have benefited from my own practice and patients, my partners, my business, and my fellow Sorry Works! Board members. And it is time to share my new learning and thoughts by revising—in a major, and, I hope, meaningful way—the first edition of *Healing Words*, for the benefit of my fellow providers and their patients.

Another change in this edition is that I have intentionally, in many instances, used the word *provider* instead of *physician*. I did this because the reality in health care is that more and more nonphysicians provide definitive medical care and/or advice, and there is no sign this trend is slowing. As a consequence, like physicians, they are directly on the front lines, so this information is clearly relevant to them. Further, use of the word *provider* is intended to include nurses, pharmacists, aides, and any others who are in the position to directly affect patient care, and who, like us all, are fallible. This book is for all of us.

The essence of the first edition of *Healing Words* remains, and the Four "R"s are alive and well, although I've added a fifth "R," encouraging providers to *remain engaged* with their patients. What has been added is additional perspective on *why* people sue and how a proactive individual can avoid ever allowing a patient to get to the point of wanting a pound of physician flesh. Transparent communication is presented as a critical factor in establishing and maintaining individual as well as organizational credibility, and such transparency creates an honesty dividend.

Indeed, in medicine, reconstructing the events leading up to an adverse outcome is a process commonly called *disclosure*. Unfortunately, that term has negative connotations in society at large, where it's used to describe the revelation of sordid—or at least unflattering—personal information. For this reason, I prefer to use the phrase *statement of transparency*, which reflects honesty, openness, and a proactive willingness to share information with patients—including details that may not shine a flattering light on the health care provider. From this point on, when you see the phrase *statement of transparency*, keep in mind that I'm referring to disclosure.

A chapter has been added on the difference between apology and disclosure, and emphasizes that either of these in isolation is insufficient to maintain the provider-patient relationship. They are inseparable; both must occur. I suggest that the *intent* behind offering apology and disclosure is no less important than the difference in intent between a surgeon and a thief holding a knife. Each is an individual with a knife, but how they intend to use it is very different.

The chapter "Our Need for Apology" has been expanded, incorporating the data that actually support the public's desire to hear the words *I'm sorry*. The chapter "The Five 'R's of Apology" has been revised. *Remedy* has been split into two components: educational and financial. Each of these is discussed with new perspective.

And I've added a fifth "R": to remain engaged. "Remain Engaged" is a chapter emphasizing that apology and disclosure are not something that one does at a single point in time and then leaves the room with everything "all better." Patients are often terrified of being abandoned by their provider after an unexpected outcome, and it is important that the provider emphasize he or she will "be there" for the patient until his or her recovery is complete.

A new chapter, "The Evidence That *I'm Sorry* Works," provides detailed information on the success of apology and disclosure programs, including true return on investment data. Information is provided to help believers overcome critics of apology and disclosure.

"Building a Culture of Civility" is the final new chapter, devoted to convincing the reader that if an organization focuses on creating civil relationships between physicians, nurses, and all staff, including apology for the least infraction, the cultural fiber of the organization changes. Patients witness the staff's respectful treatment of each other, and when they then receive an apology—whether for a cold hospital dinner or a horrific unexpected outcome—it is believable and congruent with the visible organizational culture.

The beauty of apology and disclosure is that by doing the right thing, individuals and organizations reap many *positive* unintended consequences—things that *naturally ensue*—such as enhanced communication effectiveness, improved staff relationships, lower liability because of enhanced provider-patient relationships, and, I would argue, increased patient safety. And it doesn't require you or your organization to wait for a legislature to pass a law or a medical malpractice company to give its blessing. In the vein of Nike, Just Do It!

CHAPTER 1
Reclaiming Good Medicine

"When a patient has a bad medical result, the doctor has to take time to explain what happened, and to answer the patient's questions—to treat him like a human being. The doctors who don't are the ones who get sued." It isn't necessary, then, to know how much a surgeon operates in order to know his likelihood of being sued. What you need to understand is the relationship between that doctor and his patients.
> —Malcolm Gladwell in the *New York Times* best seller, *Blink*.
> Little, Brown and Company, © 2005.

Perfection not being of this world, however, apologies remain one of the most valuable resources of the fair and considerate.
> —P. M. Forni in *Choosing Civility: The Twenty-Five Rules of Considerate Conduct*.
> St. Martin's Griffin, © 2002.

I'm sorry is one of the most commonly used phrases in any language. Few others are applicable to such a wide range of situations. The simple apology is, in fact, something of a rhetorical catchall. It's spoken as a simple act of courtesy when reaching across another person for salt at the dinner table. It's presented as a plea to judges before sentencing is pronounced. It's offered as an expression of sympathy to the bereaved.

For most people, *I'm sorry* is spoken almost reflexively throughout the day to express respect, regret, or compassion.

9

Depending on the situation and the way it's said, an apology can be everything from a throwaway social nicety to a profound utterance from the heart.

Yet for us physicians, the words *I'm sorry* are among the hardest to utter. In our profession, they are fraught with serous ramifications and nuances that other people never have to consider. In many ways, they are words that separate us from the rest of the human race.

During our training, we are taught that we must be infallible—that we cannot make mistakes. Our educations drill into us that data are absolute and that facts allow us to explain outcomes in a linear, logical fashion and figure odds with some measure of precision. It creates the expectation that if we give a patient with condition "A" medication "B," the outcome will always be "C." But no matter how much comfort we take in the scientific method, the simple truth remains that life is DUN: dynamic, unpredictable, and nonlinear. Chaos theory demonstrates that the possibility always exists for unintended consequences. Thus, our schooling sets us up to deny the failure that is embedded in our discipline, and, in fact, all of life.

> *The simple truth remains that life is DUN: dynamic, unpredictable, and nonlinear.*

Insurers and defense attorneys tell practitioners that an apology might be interpreted as an admission of fault or negligence that could expose us to litigation. Some insurers will even void the policy of a physician who apologizes to a patient in the wake of a complication or error.

CHAPTER 1
Reclaiming Good Medicine

So it's not surprising that the culture of medicine has evolved to be apology avoidant. I propose that the health care profession should take a fresh look at apology—why it is important, how to recognize when it is needed, and how it should be delivered. All of this must be examined within the context of *authentic apology**—that is, apology that is heartfelt and offered because it is the right thing to do—and not apology as a technique to manipulate and placate an angry patient to avoid a lawsuit.

As healers, we must also recognize that apology is good medicine with amazing restorative powers. We must reclaim our right to say *I'm sorry*, because we owe it to our patients. They have a fundamental human need to hear an apology when something goes awry, whether it was directly caused by us or not. In the wake of a bad outcome, saying *I'm sorry* could be as helpful for the patient's—and the physician's—psychic healing process as antibiotics are for curing an infection. This simple but eloquent phrase of compassion is as essential to a doctor's medicine bag as the stethoscope and tongue depressor.

Ironically, despite the warnings of some insurers, data indicate that the likelihood of a lawsuit falls by 50% when an apology is offered and the details of a medical error are disclosed immediately.[1] Considering our profession's urgent need to protect itself from medical malpractice liability and considering the near-anarchy over tort reform to limit jury awards, you'd think doctors would be eager to adopt a risk management strategy that offers a 50% reduction in litigation.

---

* The term *authentic* throughout this book means congruence between our inner and outer selves. The result is increased credibility and trusting relationships.

Unfortunately, medicine's difficulty with apology is symptomatic of a much larger communication crisis in health care. The environment in which physicians operate today—both literally and figuratively—makes it difficult for us to maintain our focus on the very reason we entered the field in the first place: to serve humanity. We begin learning detachment from the moment we begin medical school, and that attitude is reinforced by a system that demands practicing physicians to see more patients in less time and to be wary of engaging with them in honest, open dialogue. That's unfortunate, because the quality of our communication with patients affects every aspect of the care we provide. And it has a direct bearing on our job satisfaction as well. As P. M. Forni observes, life is a relational experience; the quality of our life depends on the quality of our relationships with others.

Reference

1. Witman A.B., Park D.M., Hardin S.B.: How do patients want physicians to handle mistakes? *Arch Intern Med* 156:2565–2569, 1996.

CHAPTER 2
A Case of Failing to Say *I'm Sorry*

Indeed, if you think of it, an apology is the payment of moral debt. That's why we say, "I owe you an apology."
—P. M. Forni in *Choosing Civility: The Twenty-Five Rules of Considerate Conduct.*
St. Martin's Griffin, © 2002.

She was an extremely fit, slender, 24-year-old female who presented with classic symptoms of appendicitis: pain in the lower right abdomen, nausea, fever, and an elevated white blood count. After obtaining informed consent, I took her to the OR to do an exploratory laparoscopy, expecting it to result in a laparoscopic appendectomy. Because I was operating in a teaching hospital, I allowed a third-year surgical resident to make the umbilical incision—not an unusual degree of responsibility for his position. His technique was not perfect, and after inserting the laparoscope, what we saw would make the heart of any surgeon skip a beat: an abdomen filling with blood from an injured artery.

We quickly converted to an open surgical procedure by making a full incision. A vascular surgeon soon arrived and controlled the accidental puncture wound with two stitches. We explored the patient's abdomen to ensure no other injuries had occurred, then performed the appendectomy and closed. Afterward, I spoke candidly with the family about what had happened, telling them this was obviously not a planned outcome or result. The patient had a rough couple of days, and I had to admit her into the intensive care unit. Her hospital stay lasted nine days.

During follow-up visits, the patient was very concerned about the scar, despite the fact that it was healing fine—from my point of view. I offered to refer her to a plastic surgeon. On the third and final follow-up visit, she complained that her "insides felt all jumbled up." Because this was a nonspecific complaint from a scientific standpoint, I dismissed it with the simple reassurance that it would get better with time. I said she could call me with questions any time and discharged her from my care.

The next time I heard from her, it was in the form of a malpractice suit. I was incredulous! How could she do this when I had saved her life? After much discussion with my attorney and malpractice insurer, we decided to fight the case. I was delighted that we were going to "defend and deny" this claim. If I'd had any idea what was to come, I would not have been so gleeful.

The legal depositions began months after the actual events. As I grew increasingly anxious about the suit, I began to see my patients in a much different light than before. I perceived each one as a possible adversary. I began habitually working out strategies for defensive recordkeeping in my head, so I would be in an advantageous position in the event of another suit. My job was no longer about care; it was about defense. It was no longer about trust and open discussion with patients; it was about cautious commentary and limiting my exposure to risk.

The next time I heard from her, it was in the form of a malpractice suit. I was incredulous! How could she do this when I had saved her life?

On the first day of the trial, my retired parents, brother, several friends, and partner attended to provide moral support. I needed it. My introduction to trial law began with 45 minutes of opening arguments in which the plaintiff's counsel derided me for incompetence as well as disregard for truth and patient welfare. He told jurors that I had committed fraud and breached my duty as a physician. He didn't merely question my character, he annihilated it. By the end of the opening arguments, my head was reeling.

The plaintiff—my patient—testified to all sorts of things regarding her care, but it was her response to the question of why she had sued that absolutely floored me: "*I sued because he acted like what happened to me was no big deal. One time when I saw him in the office after this happened, he actually put his feet up on the desk while we talked. He just didn't care.*"

That comment hit me like the heat from a blast furnace. It wasn't the injury and outcome that had led to that miserable day in court—it was her *perception* that I didn't care. My actions had communicated apathy, and that was what had landed me in court, not the medical complication.

After two weeks of intense legal debate, we won the case. Although we prevailed in battle, I still felt as if I'd lost the war. The emotional trauma of the ordeal lingered long after the case was closed. My most difficult memory surrounding the event was the reaction of my father, a physician who had practiced for more than 40 years without a single malpractice claim and the man I admire more than anyone else on earth. While my attorneys were congratulating each other, he approached me and said, "I love you with all my heart, Mike, but if you ever have to go through this again, I will not be here. I will never again willingly listen to people talk about one of my children as they have talked about you these past two weeks. It is the hardest thing I have ever done, so please don't ever ask me to do this again."

What did I learn from all this? I think the entire experience made me begin to ponder exactly how and when the entire medical profession had lost a very basic form of human kindness: the ability to offer a heartfelt, authentic *I'm sorry.*

CHAPTER 3
Anger in the Driver's Seat

When you get down to the nitty-gritty, it's the personal touch that matters.
—R. G. Sheppard, M.D., general surgeon (retired),
Smith Center, Kansas

We seem so puzzled sometimes, yet it really is quite simple, as Dr. Sheppard reminds us. It really just all boils down to the *quality* of the relationship.

When we have run out of medicines to prescribe, when there are no more surgeries we can offer, when technology has failed to provide a cure, it is just two human beings sitting together face to face, helping each other deal with the realities of life: the patient and the individual responsible for providing his or her care. And if one knows how to empathize, how to be fully present, how to be a fellow human being, in the end, that is what people really care about, especially in dire situations. Being a provider of health care has, from the very beginning, been first and foremost about caring.

Being a provider of health care has, from the very beginning, been first and foremost about caring.

It is unfortunate, then, that malpractice claims are so prevalent, because it must surely be a sign that our patients are not feeling cared for despite being treated. If, in the truest sense, they felt cared for, we would not see the frequency of litigation that we see. I challenge anyone to point to a claim in which the patient would say he or she was well cared for, either physically or emotionally. And if negligence accounts for only 17% of claims,[1] then it stands to reason that the emotional component of caring is driving the other 83%. And the emotional component driving the filing of claims is the patient's *anger*.

Quality Relationships

In 1993 Wendy Levinson, M.D., and her colleagues designed a research study they hoped would show a link between physician-patient communication and the risk of malpractice. They analyzed audiotapes of routine office visits with two groups of physicians: those who had never been sued and those with two or more malpractice suits filed against them.

Levinson found that the physicians with the best communication skills were also those who had not been sued. The former tended to ask more questions, encourage patients to talk about their feelings, use humor when appropriate, and educate patients about what to expect during treatment. These physicians also spent more time per visit with patients than those who had been sued. In fact, the length of office visits alone was strongly correlated with a physician's history of malpractice claims. How much extra time, on average, did the doctors who had never been sued spend with their patients? Three minutes.

Another group of physician researchers studied transcripts of legal depositions given by patients who had filed lawsuits. All the transcripts included the question *Why are you suing the doctor?* The study concluded that 71% of the patient-plaintiffs had had problematic relationships with their physicians before the incidents prompting the lawsuits. The researchers also identified four distinct factors underlying the suits:

1. The patients believed that their doctors had deserted them (abandonment).
2. The patients believed that their doctors had discounted their concerns.
3. The patients believed that their doctors had not provided adequate information.
4. The patients believed that their doctors did not understand their (or their families') perspectives.

Some of the most dramatic evidence revealing the effect of the patient-doctor relationship on malpractice claims comes from Gerald Hickson, M.D., and his research group at Vanderbilt University Medical Center. They set out to examine the association between unsolicited complaints about a physician, as recorded by Vanderbilt's patient affairs office, and that same physician's malpractice experiences. The authors concluded that a relatively small number of physicians generated a disproportionate share of complaints. They also found that a history of numerous complaints was an indicator that a physician runs a higher risk of being sued. In their words:

> Results are consistent with previously published research on the relationship between patients' dissatisfaction with care and malpractice claims. Patients who saw physicians with the highest number of lawsuits were more likely to complain that their physicians would not listen or return telephone calls, were rude, and did not show respect.

> Risk [of being sued for malpractice] seems not to be predicted by patient characteristics, illness complexity, or even physicians' technical skills. Instead, risk appears related to patients' dissatisfaction with their

> *physicians' ability to establish rapport, provide access, administer care and treatment consistent with expectations, and communicate effectively.*

Our Circle of Control®*

Doug Wojcieszak, the founder of Sorry Works!,† and I were doing a tag-team presentation on apology and disclosure in San Francisco at a national medical meeting when he said something, while thumping his chest with his index finger, that hit me as if he were thumping *my* chest: "I [the patient] am the driver of medical malpractice suits." I am sure if someone had been watching me closely, he or she would have been concerned that some stray spirit had just inhabited me, resulting in my dumbfounded expression. In a single sentence, much of what I had been trying to say to physicians, health care organizations, and insurers for nearly 10 years became crystal clear. And like so many things, the simplicity was brilliant.

Doug had the audacity to say that *patients* were the drivers of malpractice, not ambulance-chasing plaintiff attorneys, not poorly run medical malpractice insurance companies and their ineffectual risk management strategies. This is a unique and insightful observation for perhaps initially unapparent reasons. First, the relationship with the patient is in the provider's *circle of control*. We are in *direct* contact with the patient and can directly affect the quality of the relationship. Providers can focus on the patient beginning today. Second, lawsuits don't occur because patients are litigious. It isn't because they are greedy. It is because they are *angry*. They are angry about how the provider and the health care organization treated

---

* Registered trademark, Stephen R. Covey.
† http://www.sorryworks.net.

them. They are angry about being stonewalled when they asked questions—what? why? how?—in the aftermath of an unexpected outcome. And because they do not get answers from the people who can most directly provide this remedy, they seek answers through the only channel that remains open to them: the legal system.

Generally speaking, it is not a leap to say that the American public has a, shall we say, disdain for lawyers. As a rule, we don't like them, until, of course, we need them. With that perspective, imagine how angry or exasperated people must be to call a malpractice attorney to help them get the answers they not only seek, but deserve. The bald-faced fact is that plaintiff attorneys would have no business without angry patients and families. When patients get so angry as to call an attorney, they want answers, a bucket-o-blood, *and* money. While there will always be unscrupulous individuals who simply see a claim as their winning lottery ticket, and an attorney who will happily take the case (both issues are in the provider's *circle of concern*®,* and not in his or her control), I must believe that most claims emanate from reasonable, if not nice people who are at the end of their rope. And they are at the end of their rope because we, as providers, have failed to maintain a trusting relationship through respectful, empathetic, *transparent* communication at a time when they have a significant, emotionally driven need for information and support.

Doug developed his insight because he has been the angry family member, stonewalled by physicians and the hospital. Here is his story.

---

* Those things we are concerned with, but have no ability to affect or change. Registered trademark, Stephen R. Covey.

Doug's Story*

My brother Jim died of medical errors in May 1998. He went to a Cincinnati, Ohio, hospital at 2 A.M., complaining of chest, shoulder, neck, and stomach pains. These pains were so severe they woke him up and led him to go to the hospital. My brother was a real tough, macho guy—the kind of guy who was asked to play football in high school. He didn't go to the doctor's office or hospital at the drop of a hat. The pain that drove him to the hospital early that morning was real. However, the attending physician in the emergency department informed Jim that, at 39 years old, he was too young to be having a heart attack. This proclamation was made without drawing blood or doing an EKG. The physician, in the face of classic symptoms, did nothing to rule out the worst-case scenario for a young man, who, by the law of averages, had not yet lived half his life. They diagnosed him with stomach flu and sent him home, literally, with two Tums.

The next morning my parents had to drive Jim back to the hospital because, by that time, he was passing out due to low oxygen in his blood. This time the hospital drew blood. Sure enough, the enzyme showing the heart was in distress was present.

Jim was admitted to the ICU where the second series of errors happened. The computer monitor over his bed read, "Ray Wojcieszak." Ray is my dad's name, and my father had had heart checkups done in the very same hospital a few months before Jim's death. My dad is in his 70s, but in perfect shape—low cholesterol and no indication of heart disease. The attending physician actually argued with my father about who was whom. Ultimately, my father had to pull out driver's licenses to prove he was Ray and the man in the bed was Jim. They finally changed the computer monitor to read "Jim," but we believed it screwed up their diagnosis. Jim was diagnosed with a

---

* Adapted from personal communication with Doug Wojcieszak. Used with permission.

bacterial infection of the heart. We suspect that they had Jim's blood test of that day showing the heart in distress, but were probably looking at my father's previous charts documenting a near flawless cardiac workup. Jim's autopsy showed that he had two to three heart attacks while in the hospital under the care of his physicians.

Jim was admitted on Monday and died on Thursday. For three days, they plugged him full of antibiotics for a nonexistent infection. Day by day, he got progressively worse. On Thursday afternoon, Jim was spitting up blood, and a nurse excitedly rushed into his room and announced, "We're finally going to do something for him!" My parents, who were in the room at the time, were shocked. "Finally do something?" they wondered.

Jim was wheeled to a different room and had a probe run up his leg to check his heart. The test found three major arteries more than 95% blocked. Worse, Jim crashed on the table during the test. His finger tips and ear lobes were turning blue as he was wheeled into emergency open-heart surgery, a resident sitting on his chest pumping away to keep him alive.

Once in surgery, they were able to get him on the heart-lung machine, but they were never able to get him off the machine. The back of his heart was blown out. The surgeon who operated on Jim— who had not been involved in his care until emergency surgery was required—went to my father immediately after the surgery and said, "If these jerks at this hospital had got your boy to me three days ago, I could have saved him, no problem. It would have been a simple bypass surgery, and he would have had a long, healthy life. He's dead. I'm sorry."

The surgeon's comments were the last bit of honesty and candor we received from the hospital. After the funeral, my parents went back to the hospital seeking answers. To make a long and painful story shorter, the hospital and physicians slammed the door in their face. Even the surgeon who was so honest the night of Jim's death told my parents that hospital legal counsel had instructed him not to speak with them. This slap in the face made my parents even more angry. It made litigation, which should have been the last recourse, the only option available for answers and justice. It made money, which had been a nonissue for us, the only issue worth fighting over.

After a year and a half of litigation in very conservative Cincinnati—not a judicial hellhole by any stretch of the imagination—the judge turned to the attorneys representing the hospital and physicians and told them malpractice was clear and they needed to talk to our family. So they attempted to assuage us with some insulting offers, actually angering the judge. Only then did they offer a reasonable settlement, which we accepted. Money exchanged hands, we signed off on the settlement, and the legal battle ended. But our pain will last a lifetime.

The attorneys—not the doctors—apologized after the settlement, when there was no longer any risk to them. To our dismay, they never admitted any fault or acknowledged that they might do things differently in the future.

We believe they learned nothing from the mistakes that killed Jim, and these same mistakes could be killing other patients in their hospital and other hospitals. It's truly maddening and upsets all of us to this day. After all, no parent ever wants to bury his or her child.

Doug's story is repeated, with different circumstances and different people with different names in different cities all over the country, thousands, if not hundreds of thousands of times a year. The commonalities between the stories are too consistent to be chance, and the recurrent themes are patient and/or family anger resulting from a lack of information, disrespectful treatment, and feelings of abandonment. Time and time again, we see patients' loved ones merely desiring information and a heartfelt apology, and yet the medical, legal, and insurance industries continue to debate how to handle unexpected outcomes and medical errors.*

Time to Commit to the Obvious

Most ailing organizations have developed a functional blindness to their own defects. They are not suffering because they cannot resolve their problems, but because they cannot see their problems.

—John Gardner[†]

Why is it so hard to commit to the obvious? In the face of overwhelming evidence, why do people, entire organizations, and even industries continue to use ineffective strategies, limiting their effectiveness and inhibiting their success?

Examples are everywhere and can be seen daily by simply looking around. The funniest one I have witnessed lately, along with millions of other people, is the popular TV show *American Idol.* For those who don't know about this reality show, it is a competition of young singers. Each season thousands of people try out for a spot on the show. The first several episodes of each season, and arguably the most entertaining, are devoted to showcasing some of the best, as well as some of the worst, tryouts. It is a fascinating study in a failure to commit to the obvious.

---

* For more personal stories about medical error, the desire for apology, and understanding what happened, see http://www.sorryworks.net/article3.phtml (accessed Jun. 22, 2006).

† Quoted in *The Eighth Habit: From Effectiveness to Greatness* by Stephen R. Covey. Franklin-Covey Co. © 2004.

Every person who tries out, perhaps with the exception of a few practical jokers, really believes he or she has a chance at winning the competition. Even the most casual observer can see, however, that many of these people aren't merely lacking the talent to sing . . . they are utterly devoid of anything resembling skill. Even when the judges, who are, on occasion, brutally unkind, tell the performer that he or she stinks, individuals leave angry because "You just don't know talent when you see it." There is a complete lack of insight as to their actual skill level. It isn't just organizations that develop functional blindness.

It is time health care organizations and physicians recognize their functional blindness as it relates to the importance of authenticity, honesty, transparency, and effective communication in delivering care and maintaining the physician-patient relationship. It is important when establishing the relationship and even more important when unexpected things happen.

The medical profession has blamed the medical malpractice problem on patients and the litigious society, ambulance-chasing plaintiff attorneys, and a broken legal system. It's the easy way out, because, if that's what one believes, it relieves one of the responsibility of doing anything for themselves . . . being proactive. Unfortunately, such beliefs are not supported by reality. The reality is that health care providers have a way to *directly* and *immediately* correct the problem—by focusing on their relationship with patients and families and effective, respectful, and transparent communication. To ignore this fact is to abdicate responsibility for what happens to you to other people, which is perhaps the most disempowering, demoralizing thing I can imagine. It is time for our entire profession to commit to this obvious truth.

References

1. Localio A.R., et al.: Relation between malpractice claims and adverse events due to negligence: Results of the Harvard Medical Practice Study III. *N Engl J Med* 325:245–251, 1991.
2. Adapted from personal communication with Doug Wojcieszak. Used with permission.

CHAPTER 4
The Transparency Quotient

Even with its inherent risks—such as appearing weak, incompetent, or otherwise less than perfect—confessing mistakes signals courage, accountability, and humility. Indeed, mistakes are an opportunity to visibly demonstrate a commitment to honesty. And handling mistakes with a high degree of responsible transparency helps build a leader's reputation of credibility.
—Barbara and Elizabeth Pagano,
The Transparency Edge. McGraw-Hill, © 2004.

Health care providers and their organizations, particularly hospitals, have an image problem. Many patients assume that if something goes wrong, they will not find out about it from their doctor. This perception is driven, unfortunately, by what is assumed to be general experience, driven by highly publicized cases. (Imagine the effect Doug's story would have had on the average newspaper-reading individual if it had been a front-page story!) And a tragic consequence is that all providers become guilty by association. If you are a doctor, you are suspect. Sadly, this perception may be more accurate than we would like to admit.

Being forced to confess is a great deal different than willingly and proactively offering information.

Being forced to confess is a great deal different than willingly and proactively offering information. One must surely understand the lunacy of attempts to cover up or avoid addressing a bad outcome from a patient or family, whether or not it was the result of a medical error. People are not ignorant about what is going on with their bodies. The vast majority of the time, when something is wrong with a patient's body after some treatment, you can't hide it or convince them that everything is OK. Tiptoeing around the obvious can, and almost surely will, backfire. Doctors, nurses, and other providers, with full and enthusiastic support *and training* from their organization and insurer, should address issues head on and with complete transparency. Using down-to-earth, nontechnical language, providers should always be honest with patients and their families.

Angry and a Long Way from Home

It was 5 P.M. on Friday night, and my cell phone rang. I was on call for trauma surgery, and a critically injured patient was en route to the emergency room, having been in a T-bone type car crash. The driver's side of the car was shoved half way to the passenger's side of the car. Just getting the patient out of the crumpled car took an hour in freezing temperatures.

Remarkably, the patient, who was just traveling through Santa Fe, had few apparent serious injuries. CT scans did not show any bad injuries to internal organs. She had a small laceration of a kidney. *The spleen was specifically noted to be normal.* She had a stable fracture of the pelvis, and she required admission for pain control and observation.

Nothing, however, would be simple with this patient. The patient was a chronic alcoholic ("a couple of drinks a day"), which she neglected to mention, and she had smoked for 50 years. She soon developed alcohol withdrawal. She deteriorated and was placed on a ventilator. Her blood count (hemoglobin) dropped to about 8 gm/dl (normal being 12 to15), which I interpreted as being consistent with her kidney injury and visibly bloody urine. I gave her two units of blood, and her blood count came up to 10. She was rock stable for two days; then she had another precipitous drop in her hemoglobin, this time to 6. Another physician involved in the case gave her three units of blood, unbeknownst to my surgeon partner who was covering for me during this time over the weekend.

When my partner saw the patient several hours later, he immediately ordered a CT scan, which revealed a ruptured spleen. He took her to the operating room and removed a shattered spleen. She also developed a collapsed lung during surgery, which required a tube in her chest. Her lung most likely collapsed because of her emphysema and the rupture of a bleb (a "bubble" of lung tissue), a condition often found in long-time smokers. Needless to say, she was critically ill, and going through alcohol withdrawal to boot.

Family descended on the hospital like bald eagles during the annual salmon run. They weren't your typical family, either. One daughter was a nurse, and one was a respiratory therapist. A son was a flight instructor.

On Monday morning rounds, the ICU nurses caring for the patient informed me that the family was angry and increasingly aggressive with the staff. They wanted a meeting with all physicians involved, and they were voicing clear displeasure with their mother's care. As providers often hear, the family claimed they "didn't know what was going on. No one is talking to us." They wanted to know why the spleen injury was missed. They accused the surgeon of causing the collapsed lung. They denied their mother was alcoholic, despite the son having told us directly. They were, in no uncertain terms, angry.

Because I was the admitting physician, and the majority of her problems were surgical, I arranged for the meeting. I was aware of their concerns, so I printed copies of the admission CT scan that clearly demonstrated an *uninjured* spleen on admission, and the follow-up scan four days later showing the ruptured spleen.* These same scans illustrated her advanced lung disease, with multiple blebs, and no preoperative collapse of the lung. I printed the lab reports, by date, to show them the drops in her blood count, its subsequent stability over two days, and another drop. My intent was to be completely transparent with this angry group of people. And it worked.

Accompanied by a case manager, I presented all the information to the family. We each witnessed their anger drain right out through their feet, never to return during her nearly month-long hospitalization.

Transparent communication with this family—merely providing them with information that was rightly theirs to know—eliminated their anger and reduced their anxiety about the care their mother had and was receiving. They went out of their way to tell us how pleased they were with their mother's care.

Your Transparency Quotient†

How well do you personally handle situations in which a mistake has been made, whether or not you played some role in actually causing the mistake? Use the following mini-survey to assess how well you function in situations in which an error has caused

---

* Delayed rupture of the spleen after a traumatic accident is a rare, but recognized complication.

† Adapted from *The Transparency Edge. How Credibility Can Make or Break You in Business*, pp. 134–135. Barbara and Elizabeth Pagano. © 2004 by Barbara Pagano. McGraw-Hill, New York, NY. Used with permission.

a problem or there has been an unexpected outcome. It also indicates your civility in responding to errors.

Rate each expectation in two ways:
1. How well do you think you are doing at meeting the expectations listed in Column 1?
2. What might others think about how well you are meeting the expectations listed in Column 2?

SCALE: 1 = significant improvement needed
2 = slight improvement needed
3 = skilled/competent
4 = talented
5 = outstanding: a role model

Expectation	COLUMN 1 How do you think you are doing?	COLUMN 2 What might others think?
Willingly admits his or her mistakes.	1 2 3 4 5	1 2 3 4 5
Treats mistakes as opportunities for learning and positive change.	1 2 3 4 5	1 2 3 4 5
Effectively apologizes in a timely and sincere manner.	1 2 3 4 5	1 2 3 4 5
Forgives others' mistakes and does not hold a grudge.	1 2 3 4 5	1 2 3 4 5
Avoids blaming others.	1 2 3 4 5	1 2 3 4 5
TOTALS		

Total the points for each column. The sum of Column 1 reflects your perception of your effectiveness in handling the aftermath of errors.

22–25 points: You are doing an excellent job. You are meeting others' expectations for handling mistakes. This is what all providers should strive to achieve.

19–21 points: You need improvement in your approach to handling mistakes.

Less than 19 points: You are in a dangerous area. Your credibility may be in jeopardy. Get help now!

Next, subtract the sum of Column 2 from that of Column 1. If there is a gap of 6 points or more between how you think you are doing, and how others think you are doing (with a lower score assigned to how others might rank your ability), it indicates your intentions are perhaps more lofty than your visible actions. If the number is negative, you may not be giving yourself enough credit in the way you handle such incidents.

For a more accurate view of how others perceive you, have your co-workers complete this short questionnaire on your behalf. If they feel they are able to be honest with you, without worrying about a negative reaction, you may well learn important things about yourself.

CHAPTER 5
Bedfellows and Intent:
Apology and Disclosure

Initially, and naively, I believed that apology was the be-all and end-all as it related to maintaining the provider-patient relationship . . . as long as an authentic apology was offered on the back end of a bad or unexpected outcome, that it would be enough, that all the good things that naturally ensue while maintaining the relationship would happen. With time it has become apparent to me that apology, while of primary importance, alone is insufficient. Apology must necessarily, *although not immediately*, be followed by providing the patient and family with details surrounding the outcome. That is, disclosure of known facts.

Two camps of thought have emerged in the debate over apology and disclosure in the past several years: those who focus primarily on apology, and those who focus primarily on disclosure. As Dwight D. Eisenhower noted, positions taken on the extremes of any debate are always wrong. The truth almost always lies somewhere in the middle.

Apology without disclosure is insufficient, as it leaves patients without the information they so strongly desire. Disclosure without apology is insufficient, as it leaves patients with the sense that the provider doesn't care—he or she has no empathy or humility. Optimally maintaining the provider-patient relationship requires *both* apology and

> *Apology without disclosure is insufficient, as it leaves patients without the information they so strongly desire.*

disclosure, and in that order. Apology should precede disclosure, as it emphasizes the intrinsic value of the relationship first.

Steve Kraman, M.D., and Richard Boothman, J.D., designed and implemented two of the best publicized and successful disclosure programs in American hospitals.[1] They have expressed concern that many individuals misunderstand full disclosure programs, especially related to apology, and that such misunderstanding has slowed the adoption of disclosure programs. I, too, am continually disappointed and confused by the medical malpractice insurance industry's aversion to novel strategies to reduce claims and modify underwriting methodologies. The debate about apology and disclosure is a prime example of such resistance. Resisters offer no data supporting the widespread, dogmatic position of apology and disclosure avoidance, a position promoted for nearly 30 years that reflects both a policy and mindset that have contributed significantly to the poor state of affairs in the industry.

Kraman and Boothman suggest that apology and disclosure programs have been inappropriately portrayed as "touchy-feely and self righteous,"[1] noting that the concept of apology and the position that it is "the right thing to do" appeals to the public and health care workers. They note:

> *However, risk management professionals, defense attorneys, and insurers are flinty, hard-edged types who see the world as a dangerous place and equate soft-hearted with soft-headed. We suspect that many people in the business of risk management have not looked much beyond the apology part. . . . We can't blame them as there is far too much attention being paid to the apology and even to disclosures.*[1]

They further note that:

> *The real key component in any successful claims man-*
> *agement program, from ours at the Lexington VA, to*
> *the successful program at the University of Michigan,*
> *to that described by Sorry Works! is competent case*
> *assessment and principled management with a back-*
> *bone . . . .*

> *At the University of Michigan and the VA hospital at*
> *Lexington (the only two hospitals to publicly air their*
> *financial outcomes), risk management is a hard-nosed*
> *system based first, on working hard to know the differ-*
> *ence between reasonable and unreasonable care and*
> *next, resolving to take advantage of no one and allow-*
> *ing no one to take advantage of you . . . .*

> *A constant litany of "doing the right thing" won't per-*
> *suade the doubters. They have to understand this as*
> *the management issue that it is. Apart from the*
> *nuances of "Sorry Works!" and other such approaches,*
> *to gain real ground we need to frame the problem and*
> *the solution in real and realistic terms.*[1]

There is no doubt that apology and disclosure work miracles in reducing claims. I agree that simply telling people it is "the right thing" to do may not change behavior much, especially in the conservative risk management industry.

Management is not needed to manage or implement apology and disclosure on the level at which it will be most beneficial—daily, in the clinical trenches. Remember, more than 80% of claims are due to poor provider-patient relationship. Because most situations with upset patients do not involve bad outcomes in which the physician is at fault, it stands to reason that the management-based approach outlined by Kraman and Boothman is not needed. Rather, training the provider to meet the patient's humanistic needs, with apology and disclosure being critical components, should be the focus. Provider leadership and structured training are needed in "how to" apologize and disclose. All the organization, management, and insurers need to do is to get out of the way and give providers the green light when they recognize an apology is due, and provide information, without attempting to micromanage the relationship. Management is needed in those few instances when there is a need to assess whether the standard of care was met on a case-by-case basis. If it wasn't, as Kraman and Boothman note, management needs to ensure that "the right thing" is done for all parties.

A Philosophical Difference

There is no doubt that a structured approach is clearly beneficial. What bothers me is the seeming *intent* of such programs. The genesis of the few successful programs out there is a genuine and appropriate concern about the malpractice environment, which is, not surprisingly, the same reason I became interested in apology. The difference between what I am promoting, and what programs like these seem to promote, is a matter of *intent*: I believe in apology and disclosure because it keeps the provider focused on the *relationship* . . . satisfying the emotional and intellectual needs of patients and their families in the aftermath of an unexpected event or medical error. I believe that "doing the right thing" is, in fact, well, the right thing. It is difficult for me to believe that appealing to the better nature of others is ever wrong. It is also apparent to me that the vast majority of situations, if appropriately handled by the provider, never require involving risk management.

CHAPTER 5
Bedfellows and Intent: Apology and Disclosure

Many programs that are "out there" have been created primarily to control risk, not necessarily because it is "the right thing" to do. If risk management (that is, claims avoidance) is the primary focus, the end goal, in essence, is to *manipulate the provider-patient relationship* to the organization's advantage, not because the patient is intrinsically important as an individual. As I have noted time and again, *risk management benefits cannot be pursued as the reason for apology and disclosure.* Rather, risk management benefits naturally ensue as a by-product of maintaining the relationship.

Risk management policies that try to choreograph what providers can and cannot say, as malpractice insurers seem interested in doing ("Whatever you do, don't say 'I'm sorry.'") is an attempt to micromanage the provider-patient relationship—to control communication—and I believe can paradoxically drive a wedge between two people at a time when it is most critical for honest, respectful, transparent communication and where apology is the norm. As long as organizations continue to treat apology and disclosure as a risk management strategy, instead of an authentic attempt to help providers maintain trust and enhance the provider-patient relationship, they will continue on their path of ineffective results. They will never maximize risk management benefits because their intent is wrong. They're trying to do the right thing for the wrong reason.

Reference
1. Kraman S., Boothman R.: *Sorry Alone Doesn't Work.* The Sorry Works! Coalition. http://www.sorryworks.net/index.phtml (accessed Jun. 22, 2006).

CHAPTER 6
Roadblocks to Apology

Many factors contribute to the problem physicians have with apology, but the most glaring is the perception that offering an apology to a patient comes with legal liability. This has created the "deny and defend" culture of medicine that I, too, was caught up in before my malpractice experience. The malpractice insurance industry and defense attorneys who represent physicians in malpractice cases created this culture, and physicians have been passive accomplices. The lawyers are prone to warning doctors that patients and families may "misinterpret" a physician's sincere attempt to show compassion or regret.

However, there are fewer data to support this assumption than its alternative—that apology is actually helpful in reducing liability. In fact, there may be thousands of instances each year in which a claim is not filed due to a physician's genuine expression of regret. Still, physicians continue to tell me that when they received a letter of complaint from a patient, their malpractice insurance companies or attorneys told them to stop any and all communication with the patient. I was, in fact, told this very thing by my insurer when I was sued.

Resistance to apology by organizations and insurers is not driven by data, but by irrational fear and anecdotal experience. I have never, ever seen anyone present any compelling aggregate data on the perceived negative effect of apology. Many insurers are publicly supportive of apology and disclosure—it's the politically correct thing to do—but behind closed doors with their physicians, they say, "Never use the words 'I'm sorry.'" And yes, I know from personal experience because I have sat through such

> *Apology has nothing to do with causation. It's about empathizing, showing concern, and being respectful.*

"training sessions." The bizarre thing is that I have seen companies in states with so-called "apology laws" make these statements.

A significant barrier to apology is a simple error in logic. Many risk managers believe, "It isn't appropriate to say 'sorry' unless something bad has happened that could have been prevented and for which the person or group making the apology is responsible."[1] This is a ridiculous position, ignoring common social rules of daily life—a risk management perversion of common knowledge justified because "health care is different." When a friend has a death in the family, I tell them *I'm sorry*, yet I didn't cause their loved one's death, nor do they interpret it in that way. Apology has nothing to do with causation. It's about empathizing, showing concern, and being respectful. Social experience tells us this is true.

Another stumbling block to apology is the medical profession's ill-conceived concept of "perfectionism." For the past 30 to 40 years, medical schools have trained physicians to believe they must make faultless decisions. People who are taught they are capable of making a perfect call every time are basically programmed to meet an unfavorable outcome with denial. They think, *"It was clearly unavoidable—an act of God for which I couldn't possibly be at fault. Why should I apologize?"*

In my book *The DEPO Principle*, I describe seven qualities that are essential to success in medicine but that are actually discouraged by medical schools and residency programs. These are summarized in the chart beginning on page 42.

CHAPTER 6
Roadblocks to Apology

Author and psychotherapist Beverly Engel has noted that individuals who have difficulty apologizing possess the following traits:

- Perfectionism
- The need to be right
- Difficulty empathizing
- A tendency to be judgmental
- A willingness to project blame onto others

It's almost uncanny how Engel's list aligns with mine. No wonder the simple words *I'm sorry* are among the hardest for doctors to say. An ordinary apology of the sort delivered routinely in the course of daily life can trip up the most skilled surgeon. It can confound medical practitioners who possess some of society's most brilliant minds. In their role as healers, doctors should be master empathizers. But the same medical training that taps so effectively into their intelligence inadvertently fosters in them a kind of anti-empathy that can undermine their performance on the job.

Defining *Professionalism*
Offering an apology after a negative outcome that might have profoundly altered the course of a patient's life should be a key component of medical professionalism. I raise this suggestion at a time when the current spotlight on *professionalism* in medicine is very intense. Not terribly focused, but certainly intense. A variety of organizations are expending energy on figuring out how best to define, characterize, categorize, and teach professionalism. It illustrates a classic tendency of the medical profession—the never-ending attempt to define everything in logical, tangible terms.

Desirable Quality	Barrier to Development
Seeking win-win solutions	From start to finish, medical students compete against each other—for acceptance into the best schools, class ranking, desirable residency slots, and so on. The system is designed to win-now out the weakest at each step of the way. As a result, it teaches doctors that it's better to win than to lose, creating a culture where competition reigns supreme over cooperation. (In contrast, MBA students are taught teamwork and interpersonal skills to prepare them for a life of leading others.)
Respect for every individual	Starting out at the bottom of the proverbial ladder, medical students are often belittled and sometimes even abused by the interns, residents, and attending physicians above them. As they advance, it's always clear that their rank within the hierarchy is based on being both superior and subordinate to different sets of people and that they'll be shown little respect from anyone who has attained a higher rank.
Personal leadership	Physicians develop a belief throughout their training that because they have a modicum of control over others—patients, nurses, etc.—they are "leaders." Yet true personal leadership, according to the model used in business and other industries, stresses the ability to foster teamwork and high-trust environments, not to issue marching orders.
Flexibility	As noted above, physicians advance through a well-established hierarchy during their educations. Hierarchies are by definition inflexible. They are based on doing things in a "command and control" manner. A reliance on hard data and skepticism of softer sciences—or of anything that isn't duplicable and empirical—also leads to a rigid attitude and narrow approach that can impede problem solving. *(continued on next page)*

Desirable Quality	Barrier to Development
Teamwork	As noted above, the "win-lose" model of medical education teaches competition over cooperation. As a result, physicians tend to value autonomy. Many are uncomfortable leading, following, or even trusting their peers. Placing a high value on winning can also lead doctors to challenge anyone who disagrees with them, creating an atmosphere of distrust.
Developing others	Working in a culture of perfectionism leads to berating rather than educating people who make mistakes. (Contrast this to business environments, where training programs are built around coaching to enhance positive behaviors.) In such a culture, feedback becomes offensive instead of instructive and constructive. It's likely to elicit defensive behavior in the recipient.
Openness	Due to their training, many physicians have trouble assessing themselves accurately and receiving constructive feedback. The narrowness of their medical education also presents problems for many doctors. Medical students are taught science almost exclusively. The liberal arts are largely excluded from their education. This tight focus results in a kind of forced social illiteracy. There's no time to learn about anything else, and the world gets a little smaller. Unfortunately, this closed-mindedness to new ideas can diminish a physician's humanity, infusing him or her with a kind of clinical detachment that hampers relationships with patients.

But I believe a precise definition of professionalism will ultimately elude us, because the concept embodies a collection of qualities that each defies definition and measure. Yet we all know when we observe unprofessional behavior. And because that's the case, wouldn't it be simpler to promote professionalism by targeting and addressing its antithesis, instead of trying to teach something that defies definition?

Medical schools and continuing education programs advocate ethics and professional standards on a regular basis; however, the profession as a whole demonstrates an unwillingness to identify and amend behaviors that may have become common practice, but are inherently unprofessional nonetheless.

Part of this reluctance is a failure to apologize when contrition is clearly appropriate. Nearly every other industry considers it not only fitting, but an important part of professionalism and good customer service to express regret and offer a suitable remedy when a client is dissatisfied.

At a seminar I once attended, I heard a definition of professionalism that I've always remembered for its simplicity and universal pertinence to a wide variety of jobs. It's actually not a definition so much as a trio of behaviors that espouse personal leadership—professionalism is simply the confluence of commitment, caring, and competence. For physicians, the importance of each of these terms may not be so self-evident. Doesn't competence in medicine entail caring? Doesn't *care* refer to the processes of examination, diagnosis, and treatment planning—all of which require clinical competence and skill?

The act of caring for someone requires more than just detached, clinical attentiveness. It requires seeing the patient as a whole person with unique needs, goals, fears, and levels of health literacy. The ability of a physician to communicate caring— through empathic words, a reassuring pat on the hand, or a compassionate look—is truly a requirement of professionalism, one that's too easily overlooked in these days of managed care, where efficiency means seeing more patients in less time and ordering fewer tests and procedures.

CHAPTER 6
Roadblocks to Apology

Apology is a key way to communicate to patients that they matter and that you care about them. So, acting in a professional manner includes offering an apology when there has been a violation of trust, an unexpected outcome, or an error. Apology is just as vital to professionalism in medicine as it is in other businesses—probably more so, considering the higher stakes involved.

The business world has internalized a truth that medicine has yet to discover and embrace: Apology isn't about money or being right or wrong—for either the buyer (patient) or the vendor (doctor). It's about the provider showing respect, empathy, and a commitment to patient satisfaction; and about those receiving the apology having the grace to see the provider as human and fallible—and worthy of forgiveness.

How We Left Our Hearts to Medicine

Medicine's myopic focus on objectivity distances doctors from their patients in harmful ways. This separation is particularly damaging when a patient is in intensive care or requires heightened and detailed attention to the medico-physical aspects of care. Patients in these situations need reassurances and hand-holding—but unfortunately it is during such critical times that physicians believe it is especially important not to become emotionally involved with them.

Not a shred of evidence supports the concept that an individual cannot be both objective and empathetic at the same time. It isn't even logical to assume that being emotionally available to a patient will adversely affect the quality or objectivity of a doctor's clinical decision making. But it is safe to assume that the effort to maintain an objective demeanor while discussing an unexpected outcome often registers as coldness and lack of caring. This is a dysfunctional posturing that serves only to distance the physician from the patient at a time when the latter's emotional need is greatest.

Medicine's skeptical attitude toward the softer sciences—psychology, sociology, cultural anthropology, and so forth—is part and parcel of the mindset that erects barriers between physicians and the people they treat. Trained in the so-called "hard" sciences (and doesn't this terminology speak volumes?), physicians tend to be cynical about subjective approaches to understanding the world. They tend to dismiss the value these other fields of study have for enriching life.

Measurable data are the altar at which we physicians worship—and, to some extent, that's with good reason. Scientific inquiry has led to medical advancements that seemed like science-fiction fantasies just a decade ago.

But outside the isolating walls of the laboratory, the routine practice of medicine cannot rely on data alone. Newtonian-linear science will explain only the scientific-technical aspects of medicine—and perhaps incompletely in the end. Hard science is silent when it comes to the humanistic-interpersonal aspects of medicine, despite the fact that most practicing physicians will acknowledge that the doctor-patient relationship is an important factor in outcome.

Sometimes what counts can't be counted, and what can be counted doesn't count.

Albert Einstein, perhaps the greatest scientific mind of the 20th century, once wrote: "*Sometimes what counts can't be counted, and what can be counted doesn't count.*" But medicine tries to pare everything down to its most elemental—cells, organs, systems. In the process, we too often forget about the person whose life depends on the healthy functioning of these components.

Our goal is to heal whole people, and surely they are much greater than the sum of their parts. Philip Anderson, the 1977 Nobel Prize winner in physics (again, someone from a stringent science with a great propensity for breaking things down into their elemental components), said:

> *The ability to reduce everything to simple fundamental laws does not imply the ability to start from those laws and reconstruct the universe. In fact, the more the elementary particle physicists tell us about the nature of the fundamental laws, the less relevance they seem to have to the very real problems of the rest of science, much less society.**

In other words, as medicine understands more and more about the human body and its ailments, it seems to drift further away from humanism and the very real needs of the individuals medicine treats. As doctors, we must stop focusing exclusively on the sterile, linear-reductionist perspective and learn how to make sound scientific judgments while remaining sensitive to patients' emotional states.

This will be difficult. But if we can do it, we'll fulfill fundamental needs of both patients and physicians, because the quality of the doctor-patient relationship not only plays a significant role in healing the patient, but also in our job satisfaction.

---

* As quoted in *Complexity: The Emerging Science at the Edge of Order and Chaos* by M. Mitchell Waldrop. © 1992.

If physical scientists such as Einstein and Anderson can see the value of the softer side of science, surely the medical profession can. Physicians must be willing to accept that some things simply can't be summarized with a number and printed on a lab report. We can't send a requisition down to the pharmacy for a STAT order of humanism, compassion, or empathy. These must come from within—not as part of a formula for "managing" a relationship, but as an authentic, heart-felt desire to recapture what the profession has lost.

Unfortunately for everyone involved, patients are likely to view physicians' well-intentioned emotional disengagement as coldness and even of lack of caring, just when they are in greatest need of reassurance and support. As patients grow dissatisfied—even angry—about this, physicians may have no idea there's a storm brewing. They may feel they are demonstrating compassion and concern for their patients through dispassionate, unflustered attention to the clinical hurdles that stand in the way of wellness. Yet not surprisingly, compassion felt by physicians is invisible to patients unless those sentiments are translated into compassionate, visible actions—a gentle touch, a caring smile, the act of really listening, and perhaps an occasional, sincere *I'm sorry*.

Reference
1. Roman K.: Not so fast with I'm sorry. *Medical Liability Monitor*, Sep. 2005.

CHAPTER 7
Our Need for Apology

No matter what role you play in health care, at one time or another you've been a consumer of medical services. You have been the patient. Try to remember the last time a doctor apologized to you, even for a relatively minor infraction such as keeping you waiting. Can you recall a single instance?

If you're a clinician, consider these questions: When was the last time you told a patient *I'm sorry*? When did you last hear another physician apologize to a patient? To a nurse? To a hospital resident? To a medical student?

Your Honor or Your Life

The concept of apology as we conceive it today has not always existed. It is, in fact, a relatively new social model. In the not-too-distant past, if you harmed or offended another person, a duel was the likely method of resolution. You would defend your honor and reputation with your life—or death. That was an accepted part of the social order.

Eventually, people came to understand that preserving your good name did not necessarily require pistols or sharp objects. As people sought new ways to resolve personal disputes and avenge insults, the practice of apology was born. (For more about the history of apology, see *Mea Culpa: The Sociology of Apology and Reconciliation* by Nicholas Tavuchis.)

Today, certain rules are widely understood by society-at-large regarding what an apology means and when it is appropriate. Even minor infractions of etiquette often elicit an apology from the offender. When you accidentally bump into another person, don't you say, "*Excuse me?*" Such an apology carries three meanings: The offender (1) shows respect for the other person, (2) shows respect for the rule that was broken, and (3) admits his understanding of the rules, and in so doing promises to abide by them in the future. Most offended people accept apologies, allowing them to preserve the relationship, reestablish trust and respect, and reenter society with their honor intact.

But physicians have been told—and have come to believe—that it is imprudent to express contrition or regret to patients in the event of an unexpected outcome. This has resulted in a sophisticated sort of social "de-evolution" in health care—in essence, a permissible and sanctioned loss of civility. As a result, physicians and patients must rely on dueling to settle disputes when the patient has been "offended," whether physically, emotionally, or both. These duels are called medical malpractice lawsuits, and they are the civilized equivalent of a battle to the death.

Like the duels of yore, these courtroom combats are absolute win-lose situations. Even when physicians prevail, they are never the same psychologically. Having been through the process, I can say with conviction that it takes a toll on one's soul. I would much rather avoid the duel entirely and defend my reputation instead through the simple, honorable act of an apology when I've somehow let down my patients. I think the day is coming when more of my colleagues will choose this route as well.

Healing the Relationship Is Proactive Risk Management

As physicians, we tend to think of healing in purely corporeal terms—broken bones knitting together, sutures closing a gaping wound, antibiotics staving off an invasion of rogue microbes.

CHAPTER 7
Our Need for Apology

But apology is also about healing. Specifically, it's about healing relationships that have been damaged by any number of means. Beverly Engel provides a compelling example in her book *The Power of Apology*, which she wrote after her estranged mother apologized to her out of the blue for the childhood emotional abuse she'd inflicted on Engel. After hearing the words *I'm sorry*, Engel recalls:

> *Waves of relief washed over me. Resentment, pain, fear, and anger drained out of me. Much to my surprise, those two simple words seemed to wipe away years of pain and anger. They were the words I had been waiting to hear most of my life.*

Tremendous restorative energies are released when our transgressors simply acknowledge the roles they have played in our pain. In medicine, apology has the power to repair a violation of trust (real or perceived) that results from an unexpected outcome, complication, or medical error. It can defuse the interest of a patient or his family in pursuing financial compensation as revenge for being wronged. I believe that a heartfelt apology can be helpful in any phase of the process, even after a claim has been filed.

When a physician apologizes authentically to a patient, the apology is likely to be received as a gift. It is reciprocated by the patient's forgiveness of the physician, the restoration of trust in the relationship, and, all things being equal, a lower likelihood of a lawsuit.

Of course, the act of contrition must be authentic if it is to have its intended healing effect. An apology offered purely as a risk management tool to avoid a lawsuit is nothing more than a manipulation and may very well backfire, making a situation worse.

As it has been used historically in health care, the term *risk management* was applied to defensive activities designed to prevent or reduce financial liability stemming from a patient's injury or adverse outcome. The problem with such activities is that they placed physicians and hospital administrators in an adversarial role with the patients they are trained to serve. Risk management, as we know it today, is struggling with its identity. Although risk management is about avoiding exposure that may lead to litigation, a growing number of risk managers recognize that the real way to reduce exposure is through respect for the patient and maintaining a trusting relationship. It will take time for that trend to take hold. In the meantime, risk management may be viewed by some as purely a financial function.

But authentic apology is entirely about healing the relationship and maintaining trust. It is driven by honor and ethics, not by financial self-protection. Still, there are plenty of data to support that tangible, fiscal rewards are a natural by-product of authentic apology.

Research shows that patients are less likely to consider litigation when a physician has been honest with them and expressed regret about mistakes or poor outcomes. Patients and family members who receive heartfelt apologies can be amazingly generous in their responses, sometimes even finding the grace to console a distraught physician. On the other hand, patients and families who are denied this outlet may choose to seek a very different means of healing. Believing that "revenge" will bring them peace, they choose litigation as a means of forcing the open and honest discussion they've been denied.

CHAPTER 7
Our Need for Apology

"We Wept Together"

The power of an honest, open relationship between a physician and a patient is illustrated by the following true story, related to me by a friend:

> One evening, as I was about to leave the office, one of my colleagues knocked on the door asking if he could see me for a few moments. As I motioned for him to sit, I could tell this was not a social visit—he appeared to be deeply troubled. After a long period of silence, he began to speak.
>
> "David, I am terribly torn about something, and I do not know what to do. I am hoping you will help me with a decision that I can't seem to make on my own."
>
> He went on to relate how, a few days earlier, he had delivered an infant who died a few hours after birth. The infant was the child of a woman he'd actually delivered 25 years earlier and had cared for during his entire practice. After describing some of the details regarding the infant's death, he quickly came to the point of his struggle: "The family sent me a funeral announcement. I don't know what to do."
>
> His dilemma came down to this: He was reluctant to do anything that would point to his personal failure in delivering this infant and potentially increase the liability of an already high-risk situation.
>
> At that point, I asked him to repeat some of the details of the delivery. "Did you actually do anything wrong?"' I asked.
>
> He replied, "I've gone through the events over and over again, and I really feel the delivery went as it should have and everything that occurred afterward was unpreventable."

Ultimately I asked, "What does your heart tell you to do?"

He said, "I really want to go to that funeral."

I told him, "Then by all means, go."

A few weeks later, we crossed paths. He motioned to me to come into his consult room. We sat down together and he said, "I just wanted to tell you what happened since I last saw you. I attended the funeral and something remarkable happened. As the service concluded and the mourners were departing, one of the family members came up to me and asked if I would stay behind so that the grieving mother and family could have a moment alone with me. As I stood hand in hand within this small circle, they told me how much it meant to them that I cared enough to be there to share this moment of grief with them. Then, we wept together."

With that, he got up out of his chair and said, "Thanks for letting me share that with you. I had better get back to my patients."

This case never ended up in the courts, and I'm convinced there was no lawsuit because this physician had established a trusting relationship with the family long before the incident in question took place. When a tragic outcome occurred, he remained grounded in caring and made himself available to the patient and family. His actions helped everyone heal—including himself.

As this story poignantly illustrates, avoiding a lawsuit isn't the only reason to apologize to a patient. It's an act that also heals the healer. Compare the narrative above with the following about a medical resident who failed to follow up on an abnormal test result—a chest x-ray that revealed the presence of a cancerous lesion in a patient's lung. The doctor didn't realize his mistake until he opened the man's chart a year later, during a routine annual checkup, and saw the forgotten progress note about the positive x-ray. He relates:

Realizing my oversight, I immediately reported it to the residency director. In the next agonizing weeks, I spoke with a psychiatrist on the faculty as well as with other residents and my advisor. I discussed the situation endlessly with my wife, recalling every detail and wondering how I could have "forgotten" such a critical detail. At the same time, I skirted the issue with the patient's son, although I indicated that something might have been done sooner. I felt the right thing to do was to tell the son the truth, but I was advised that doing so would invite a lawsuit. I felt like a moral failure.

I didn't sleep at all for three days, and then only intermittently. My progress note replayed itself endlessly in my mind. I checked in frequently with my patient to arrange chemotherapy, pain control measures, and, ultimately, hospice care. I last visited my patient two days before his death, which was five months after I uncovered my mistake. He was sleeping in a warm room in his house. His son and I watched him for a few minutes, then we hugged and I left. I will never forget this patient, and I think of him whenever I screen and examine patients, knowing that I don't want to miss another important diagnosis.*

---

* Albert W. Wu. "A Major Medical Error: Medical Resident Tells How He Coped With It." Reproduced with permission from the March 1, 2001 issue of *American Family Physician*. Copyright ©2001 American Academy of Family Physicians. All Rights Reserved.

This case illustrates how physicians all too often allow fear of litigation to deprive them of the healing powers of apology. The resident acknowledged his error to his wife, his colleagues, and his supervisor—essentially to everyone but the two people (the patient and his son) whose forgiveness might have released him from his emotional agony. He also seems to have sought comfort by becoming unusually attentive to the dying patient, personally coordinating aspects of care outside his own area and even visiting the patient and his son at their home. Yet these attempts to assuage his own guilt by somehow making it up to the patient ultimately seem to have been less effective at allowing him to "defend his honor" than a simple apology might have been.

From a risk management standpoint, if the patient or family had discovered the nondisclosure of the error, they would have felt doubly wronged and would most likely have reacted with anger. A 1992 study by Gerald Hickson, M.D., found that of 127 families who sued health care providers for perinatal injuries, 24% were motivated to litigate because they suspected or recognized a cover-up. As we'll see later, apology is best coupled with full disclosure as soon as possible after an error or unexpected outcome. This policy is slowly gaining favor among a few organizations that refer to it as "humanitarian risk management."

Regarding the anecdote about the resident above, I find it sad that this young doctor, still in a training phase of his career, didn't receive any encouragement from his teachers and role models to be open and honest with the patient and his family. It comes down once again to how we teach professionalism— is it any wonder that apology doesn't come naturally to physicians?

CHAPTER 7
Our Need for Apology

A Preponderance of Evidence— And Common Sense

There is a predominant expectation among the general public, our patient population, that apology is desired in the aftermath of a bad outcome, whether or not the outcome is directly caused by a physician. Apparently, however, many question this, despite its basis in common sense, and providers continue to be coached never to utter the words *I'm sorry*.

For this reason—that is, the common sense nature of apology, in addition to the extreme resistance in the medical malpractice insurance industry—I launched a Web-based survey regarding apology.

The goal of the poll was simple. What words do people feel constitute an apology? What do people want to hear when there has been a complication? While these data from 651 respondents probably wouldn't pass muster for publication in a medical journal, the results support the common sense approach promoted in this book.

If you had a serious or life-threatening complication during treatment by your doctor, but it was NOT his or her fault, which of the following would you like to hear from your doctor?	Percentage (%)
1. I really don't know how to tell you, but you have had a complication.	12%
2. I really wish it wasn't so, but you have had a complication.	21%
3. I am really sorry, but you have had a complication.	43%
4. I really regret it, but you have had a complication.	13%
5. I hoped I wouldn't have to tell you, but you have had a complication.	11%

By a factor of two, people would most like to hear the words *I'm sorry*, after a bad complication not caused by their physician. But what if their physician was at fault?

If you had a serious or life-threatening complication during treatment by your doctor, and it WAS his or her fault, which of the following would you like to hear from your doctor?	
	Percentage (%)
1. I really don't know how to tell you, but you have had a complication.	9%
2. I really wish it wasn't so, but you have had a complication.	7%
3. I am really sorry, but you have had a complication.	53%
4. I really regret it, but you have had a complication.	24%
5. I hoped I wouldn't have to tell you, but you have had a complication.	7%

The finding of most interest to me in these data is the relationship between a desire to hear the words *I'm sorry* and the physician's role in causation. In other words, the more direct a physician's role in having actually caused harm, the greater the desire patients have to hear the words *I'm sorry* from the physician.

Another goal of this survey was to understand what most people consider the strongest statement of apology. Of three choices, "I'm sorry this happened," was by far understood by most as being the strongest apology.

Which statement do you feel is the strongest apology?	
	Percentage (%)
1. I regret this happened.	31%
2. I'm sorry this happened.	58%
3. I wish this hadn't happened.	1%

Why is this information important? Because many organizations and medical malpractice insurance companies tell their providers (behind closed doors) never to use the words *I'm sorry*. Unfortunately, that is what most of our patients want to hear.

While much criticism can be leveled at these data, the consistency is remarkable. Further, ignore the results at your own risk. This is clearly saying *I'm sorry* matters!

My survey is bolstered by the American College of Physician Executives 2006 Patient Trust and Safety survey of more than 1,000 patients. They found that patients are nearly 60% less likely to sue a physician who apologizes after a medical error.[2] Survey respondents were, on the flip side, 92% more likely to sue a doctor who tried to hide a medical mistake. Keep in mind that nondisclosure, regardless of why, appears to a patient as "hiding a mistake." Sixty-one percent of physicians in this survey believed they would be less likely to be sued if they apologized after a medical mistake . . . three times the number of physicians who believed it increased their likelihood of being sued!

Of Human Bonding

Why do the simple words *I'm sorry* have such deep, extraordinary power to mend relationships? In her book *The Power of Apology*, Beverly Engel identifies five important messages that are communicated whenever they are spoken.

1. Apologizing to a person says you respect him.
2. Apologizing shows you are able to take responsibility for your actions.
3. Apologizing demonstrates you care about the way the other person feels.
4. Apologizing reveals you feel empathy for the other person.
5. Apologizing shows your desire to resolve anger the other person feels.

Respect, responsibility, caring, empathy, and dissipating anger are pretty strong medicine when applied to a physician and patient faced with an unexpected treatment outcome. Why?

Demonstrating Respect

A study at Vanderbilt University found that the patients of

physicians who received frequent complaints said they felt the physicians did not respect them. These patients understandably grew angry in the event of unexpected outcomes or errors, believing they received substandard care due to lack of respect. A physician who does not apologize or otherwise express regret for a complication exacerbates such a perception when it already exists. Humanistic risk management calls for establishing rapport with the patient as quickly as possible, but it's particularly critical to demonstrate empathy and respect for a patient dealing with a less-than-desirable outcome.

Taking Responsibility

When a treatment or intervention goes badly, the patient has the right to know who will be responsible. But most patients are not as interested in "responsibility" in the sense of who is to blame as they are in who will be responsible for helping them get better. A physician can—and should—assume responsibility for coordinating care, for finding out what happened and why, and for keeping the patient and family informed. Telling the patient, *"I'm sorry this has happened to you, and I want to assure you I'll continue to oversee your care,"* can immediately alleviate the patient's fear of being abandoned during a difficult time. The bottom line is that while the provider may not be responsible for causing the bad outcome, he or she is always responsible *to* the patient.

Showing Compassion

When patients experience a negative outcome, they want to believe that their caregiver is deeply concerned. An apology lets patients know that their troubles aren't being shrugged off. Patients sense caring not just in the words a physician delivers, but also in the eye contact, touch, and tone of voice that accompanies the apology.

However, physicians should strive to relate to their patients and earn their trust on an ongoing basis—not just in the event of an unfortunate mistake or unforeseen problem. The following story, related by a resident during a focus group I sponsored in Chicago on doctor-patient relationships, shows why:

> *When I was in medical school, a teacher told us of this one case that happened to one of his mentors. One of his patients died, and the doctor acknowledged that he'd made a mistake. Someone approached the patient's son about suing the doctor, but the son refused. He said, "My father loved this doctor. He felt that he could call him at home anytime, day or night, with any question. There was no such thing as a dumb question. Everyone makes mistakes, and it's not this doctor's fault that he just happened to make one bad mistake. I won't sue him for that."*

Expressing Empathy

In a series of focus groups led by physician-researcher Dr. Thomas Gallagher in 2002, participants were allowed to observe quietly and unobtrusively while several physicians discussed their experiences with medical errors. The nonphysician participants later reported feeling shocked to learn just how devastated doctors felt when their actions brought about an unintended consequence. The public seldom sees this side of doctors, because too often the urge to convey empathy to the patient is perverted by legal concerns. Yet it is a feeling that should absolutely be tapped into, as it will facilitate healing for all parties involved.

Dissipating Anger

We don't need to delve into the research literature for proof that apology dissipates anger. We simply need to recall a time when we were angry about a real or perceived transgression but decompressed when our transgressor offered an authentic apology. This is a very basic human response.

Four Motivations for Apology

I wish it were enough to simply write about the reasons apology is important. Unfortunately, many times knowing that something is important fails to inspire us to do it. In the absence of proper motivation, common knowledge doesn't always translate into common practice. For instance, my motivation to work out, change my diet, or quit smoking might be very different if I suffered a major heart attack at the age of 45.

Apologizing is like that, too. Without motivation, physicians are less likely to do it. The good news is, I believe most physicians are driven by an honorable set of ethics and morals. I think they care about their patients. And I believe the motivation to apologize has always existed, but for the variety of complex and interrelated reasons outlined above, the profession has been actively discouraged from it.

Beverly Engel identifies four basic motivations for apologizing:
1. To express regret
2. To assuage a guilty conscience
3. To salvage or repair a damaged relationship
4. To escape punishment

Let's look at each one of these as it relates to instances of unexpected outcomes in health care.

Expressing Regret
Expressing regret is the "purest" reason for apologizing. Apology

does not necessarily imply guilt or constitute a confession. If a patient is experiencing more than typical postoperative pain for a procedure, a caring physician might tell him or her, "I'm sorry you're in so much pain." Obviously, the physician is simply demonstrating empathy, not assuming culpability for the pain. Such expressions of regret and empathy build trust and forge bonds of common humanity.

Physicians are also motivated to apologize when they play a direct, causal role in an unexpected outcome. Apologies in these instances can be phrased in a way that avoids assigning blame to any one individual.

Assuaging a Guilty Conscience
When a physician is responsible for an unexpected outcome, feelings of guilt may underlie his or her apology. If that guilt is not accompanied by a healthy dose of regret, the effect could be less than desired. Assuaging a guilty conscience is a selfish motivation, and the doctor who apologizes solely so he or she can sleep at night runs the risk of coming off as a whiner who's more concerned about himself or herself than the patient's physical and emotional problems.

Preserving a Relationship
An apology is always most effective offered up front, as soon as the offending incident occurs. An apology offered later as a means of damage control is likely to be perceived as insincere. The offended party might sense the apologizer is not really sorry for what he's done but very sorry he was caught.

Risk Management
If a physician's apology seems inconsistent with his or her past behavior, the patient will regard it as a manipulative ploy to avoid

a malpractice suit. Doctors who cultivate open, honest relationships with their patients all along can avoid this perception.

The XY Factor

One reason apology is so hard for physicians is the "XY" factor. For now at least, the majority of doctors are men—and men are more likely to be raised to avoid showing signs of weakness. It's ironic, but many males seem to consider saying *I'm sorry* to be the equivalent of admitting defeat, of rolling over and showing their throats (or exposing their hearts). Due to their socialization, men also tend to be less skilled at communication, especially when it comes to discussing feelings—the infamous Mars-Venus conundrum.

On the other hand, perhaps because of their role in the family and society as nurturers, women tend to be better communicators. Thus, female physicians have greater success connecting with their patients. A study of 667 graduates of Jefferson Medical College concluded that women valued the psychosocial aspects of medical care more than males. A larger, national survey of 2,326 physicians revealed that the women felt, on average, that they needed 15% more time to provide what they considered to be high-quality care.

This indicates a greater need—and skill—on the part of female physicians to foster the doctor-patient relationship. So it should come as no surprise that yet another study found male physicians were three times more likely to be sued for malpractice than their female colleagues. As women's representation in medicine increases—and in 2004, for the first time, the number of women entering medical schools surpassed that of men—their influence should help change medicine's perception of the doctor-patient relationship in positive ways.

Reference

2006 Patient Trust and Safety Survey. *The Physician Executive*. Mar.–Apr. 2006.

CHAPTER 8
The Five "R"s of Apology

According to Beverly Engel, an authentic apology has three key elements: regret, responsibility, and remedy. In health care, a fourth and fifth must be added—one that precedes the other three: recognition of when an apology is needed, and one that follows the other three: remaining engaged with the patient.

Although knowing when to say *I'm sorry* may seem intuitive for most people, physicians, as we have discussed, are inclined to have difficulty. Medicine's emphasis on deny-and-defend risk management practices, coupled with the attitudes instilled in doctors during their training, can make apologizing actually seem counterintuitive for them.

The five components of apology—recognition, regret, responsibility, remedy, and remaining engaged—all need to be present, and preferably in that order, or else the person receiving the apology will sense that something is amiss. In fact, I believe skipping any of the components has the potential to make the situation worse—for example, expressing regret to an injured patient but failing to initiate a remedy for the harm that's been done could be infuriating.

> *The five components of apology are recognition, regret, responsibility, remedy, and remaining engaged.*

Recognition

The key to recognizing when to offer an apology is being aware of one's own feelings as well as those of the recipient. If the doctor feels regret or remorse, or senses that her relationship with the patient is on tenuous ground, these are clear internal signals that an apology may be in order. Likewise, if the patient's (or family's) body language or manner of interaction with the doctor seems strained, this can be a clue that the patient feels there are unmet expectations with regard to outcome or communication. Sometimes what patients don't say is more important than what they do, and being able to read their visual clues is critical.

Of course, in many situations it's obvious an apology is warranted, particularly when the patient is dealing with an adverse outcome. In these circumstances, the doctor must recognize that fear and uncertainty are normal reactions that can cause the patient to lash out angrily. The patient may storm in, demanding answers to questions that you simply can't address without obtaining some answers of your own first. It is critical that you do not become defensive, withdrawn, or evasive. Say that you hope to address all the questions and concerns, but first you need to know more about the situation. Ask for permission to return to the questions as soon as you've learned what you need to know in order to respond adequately.

Consider saying *"I'm sorry you're upset—I'm upset about this too. I am doing everything I can to understand how and why this happened."* If necessary, excuse yourself from the room to clarify your thoughts, gain your composure, and/or look up an answer to the patient's question. But avoid having the patient leave your office unsatisfied, even it means throwing you off schedule. That could damage the relationship—perhaps permanently—and provoke the patient to consult with an attorney before you get to the "regret" phase.

While the focus of this book is apology in the context of a

medical error or complication, I encourage you not to reserve *I'm sorry* just for mishaps. Expressions of regret are considered courteous behavior in many situations. Examples of when a physician should apologize include the following:

- Being late for a scheduled appointment
- Receiving a patient complaint about poor service from hospital or office staff
- Interrupting a patient who is speaking—even if you must take an emergency call

In the course of daily life, keep tabs on how well you recognize situations—even minor infractions—in which an apology is appropriate. Pay attention to how you use apology outside health care. Do you excuse yourself when you inadvertently offend someone? Raise your voice in frustration? Remember, professionalism is a way of life, not just something to be paraded around at work.

Regret

An expression of regret informs your patient that you recognize his or her pain, anxiety, or fear—and that you feel badly about it. In the event of an unexpected outcome (whether or not caused by error), a simple expression of regret might go something like this:

> *I really regret this has happened. I know it's not what either of us wanted or expected, and I'd like you to know how very sorry I am for what you're going through.*

This exchange should occur immediately after you discover the complication. It allows the relationship to begin healing. A full disclosure and a remedy can come later, after you've had time to fully assess the situation. That said, these two steps should not be put off for long, or else the patient and/or family may perceive the apology as incomplete.

Responsibility

This is the step of apology that keeps insurers, health care administrators, risk managers, and physicians awake at night. Bear in mind that taking responsibility does not necessarily imply acknowledging that you made a mistake. It is critical, however, that as the provider, you understand that while you may not be responsible for having caused the complication, |*you are always responsible to the patient. Never let a patient feel he or she is going through this alone.*

Responsibility includes accurately disclosing everything you know about the situation in question. The following is an example of a statement of responsibility:

> *I am responsible for your care and will find out what happened—and, if possible, why it happened. I will keep you posted of what I learn and how it can be used to prevent future errors. At this point, I'm not sure if I would have done anything differently, but I intend to explore this thoroughly.*

These statements are most effective when offered in the first person singular—"I"—rather than the first person plural, or what is sometimes called "the royal we." Substitute "we" for "I" in the example above, and you'll see how it depersonalizes the message and creates the impression that the physician is trying to deflect responsibility:

CHAPTER 8
The Five "R"s of Apology

We are responsible for your care and will find out what happened—and, if possible, why it happened. We will keep you posted of what we learn and how it can be used to prevent future errors. At this point, we're not sure if we would have done anything differently, but we intend to explore this thoroughly.

Of course, situations occur in which the physician directly or indirectly causes the problem. I am not speaking of complications due to incompetence, which are outside the scope of this book, but rather honest mistakes resulting from communication failures, technical errors due to fatigue or limited resources, or situations beyond the doctor's control, such as idiosyncratic drug reactions or unexpected anatomical aberrations. But in these situations, the physician still initiated the treatment. Regardless of how impossible the complication was to anticipate, the physician must still assume responsibility.

A statement of transparency to offer when the physician has caused the injury or unexpected outcome might be the following:

I am responsible for your care and for this regrettable outcome. The drug reaction you experienced has been reported, but it is very uncommon. I'm looking into matters to see if your reaction could have been anticipated. At this point I can't say I would have done anything differently, but I will keep you posted of what I learn.

Remedy
An authentic apology should include an offer of restitution—a remedy that corrects the error and/or prevents it from recurring. Of course, "remedy" is a dreaded word in this context. It

conjures the specter of six- or seven-figure settlements or judgments. But confronting unfortunate outcomes directly and handling them with sensitivity can defuse the outrage that fuels these outlandish awards.

Remedy has two components, *educational* and *financial*. The educational component is satisfied if the disclosure process provides information that we now understand the patient wants in the aftermath of an unexpected outcome. The financial remedy that I speak of is not a last-minute settlement on the courthouse steps just prior to the start of a medical malpractice trial. It is simply providing for the patient's immediate financial needs surrounding the event itself. Increasingly, evidence suggests that patients are not looking to spin the Wheel of Fortune. Rather they are worried about paying their rent or a mortgage, who is taking care of their dog, or if their lawn is dying.

Educational Remedy

Gallagher identifies three major questions that patients want answered following an unexpected outcome:

- What is being done to correct the problem that I now have?
- How will this affect my health in the short and long term?
- Am I going to be responsible for the cost of this error or complication?

Note that the question "Who caused this?" is conspicuously absent from this list. Each of these questions reflects the patient's need for remedy. The first two can be addressed with a statement such as the following:

I am personally going to do everything in my power to understand why and how this happened, and I will

*keep you informed about what I learn. In the mean-
time, I have ordered antibiotics that will help. While it
is still a little too early to tell, I don't think this will
result in any long-term health problems—but I'll ver-
ify that with some lab tests in a week or two. I want
you to know this problem occurred because of a communication error, and I'm already looking into making changes that will prevent this kind of error from
ever happening again.*

In a single paragraph, one has provided two of the three key elements identified as being important to patients. It isn't difficult, and nothing in the statement implies guilt. Further, as you will see later, if the educational remedy is provided, *the majority of patients will not need or request any financial support.*

As you read the statement above, it is clear that the provider will be circling back to the patient, providing updates as more information becomes available. This is a critical point: *The provider must remain engaged* throughout this process and can't become complacent. To do so—to avoid spending face time with the patient and family due to one's discomfort with the situation—may result in the patient feeling abandoned. And the sense of abandonment is a major driver of litigation. The apology and disclosure process is not a single point in time, but part of the continuum of care. I'll speak more about this in the chapter "Remain Engaged."

Financial Remedy

The statement above provides the desired educational remedy, but doesn't address who is going to pay for the cost of the error or complication. This has the potential to be sticky and very expensive, but it doesn't have to be. When a patient knows that his or her immediate costs will be covered, evidence is mounting that his or her interest in seeking revenge through punitive damages diminishes. Both the hospital and physician can waive fees for services, absorb the costs of further medical treatments, and pay for inconveniences suffered by the patient and family.

Some hospital executives and risk managers cringe at the thought of paying money to support such patient needs. The concern is that such action may suggest to the patient that there has been some mistake made by the provider or organization. Or it may be a simple issue of cost. Either way, it doesn't require a degree in accounting to understand that the costs of providing for immediate needs could be several thousand dollars. One must surely appreciate that a few thousand offered in the spirit of doing what is right will have the potential of avoiding a future claim, which, on average, costs tens of thousands of dollars. Which amount do you want to pay?

The Fifth "R"

The 4 "R"s originally stood for *recognition, regret, responsibility,* and *remedy.* A key addition to this second edition is a fifth "R": *Remain engaged.* In other words, the provider needs to appreciate the patient's need to know that the provider is there for him or her in the aftermath of an unexpected outcome. This is an important enough concept to be the subject of the next chapter.

Timing and Planning

If you have to eat crow, do so while it is hot.
—Alben Barkley, Vice President to
Harry S. Truman

An apology should be initiated as soon as possible after discovery of the infraction, error, or unanticipated outcome. Delays in communication make patients and families suspicious. We all know from our own experience that when we are owed an apology, the longer it takes to receive it, the angrier we become.

Still, physicians shouldn't be in such a hurry that they proceed without careful thought and preparation. Even when the doctor has established a good rapport and trust with the patient, a poorly delivered or ill-conceived apology could unravel the relationship, particularly in dealing with severe situations.

Engel recommends pondering six steps before offering an apology in order to avoid delivering one that's weak and ineffective. Five of those steps are relevant to health care*:

1. Admit to yourself what has happened to the patient.
2. Ponder the ramifications of the actions or inactions that led to or caused the problem.
3. Look at the situation from the perspective of the patient and try to understand what her feelings might be (anger, fear, anxiety, pain, etc.).
4. Forgive yourself for any causal role you had in the incident (real or perceived).
5. Plan and prepare your apology.

The physician should set the tenor of the discussion from the outset. To be effective, your body language must be in synch with your words and tone of voice. Imagine a doctor standing at a patient's hospital bedside with arms crossed and delivering an apology while gazing intermittently out the window or glancing at the TV. Not only would the apology seem inauthentic, it

---

* Engel's sixth point is to "forgive the other person for harm done to you in the past," advice that's not relevant in the setting addressed here.

might actually further infuriate the patient and family members. Apology must be approached with a demeanor of humility. The doctor should sit on a chair placed within touching distance and maintain appropriate eye contact. Or if the doctor sits on the patient's bed, he or she should ask the patient's permission before doing so.

Compelled Apology: Remorse on Demand

A compelled apology is one given in response to a demand, policy, or mandate. In general, there are three groups that may call for a doctor's apology: the patient, the patient's family, or a health care organization administrator. (I should add that I've personally seen a nurse or two demand that a physician apologize to a patient's family.) Requests for an apology that come from a hospital, clinic, or insurance administrator are often precipitated by a complaint they've received—a complaint that has them concerned about exposure.

The most critical advice I have for a fellow physician caught in this situation is not to respond immediately. A demand for an apology can feel like an ambush, especially if the doctor was not previously aware of the problem. Avoid the pitfall of giving a knee-jerk, defensive response. If you need time to prepare an answer, then ask for it:

> *I see that you are angry. I would like a few minutes to reflect on my performance and how it has led to the current situation. Let me think this over so I can respond thoughtfully and accurately to your concerns and offer an appropriate apology.*

A note of caution: If you use this approach and tell patients or family members that you'll return in a few minutes, keep your promise. Don't return 20 minutes or half an hour later. They will probably be watching the clock, and your tardiness could be perceived as yet another violation of trust. It may be all that's needed to provoke them into calling an attorney.

From what I've observed, the filing of a claim often is not triggered by an isolated incident, but rather by a consistent pattern of small violations of trust and insensitivity that were tolerated until the proverbial final straw landed on the camel's back. In other words, a patient who seems suddenly to have turned on you—who is standing in your office and angrily demanding an apology—might have been dissatisfied for a while. Now he's finally venting his pent-up ire and frustration over what might seem like a relatively minor infraction. Physicians can avoid these situations by making it a habit to always treat their patients with honesty and respect, including offering apologies when they are in order rather than waiting until they are ordered.

So, what if you take the time out to ponder the situation and simply cannot figure out what the patient or family is angry about? What if you don't know what you're being asked to apologize for? Be honest:

> I appreciate the time you gave me to reflect on things. I understand you are angry, but I am embarrassed and upset to admit that I am not sure what you are angry about. Help me understand your perspective, so I can make things right by you and ensure that I don't make the same mistake again.

In this scenario, not only does the physician recognize the patient's disappointment, but also asks for the patient's help in understanding the situation. This scenario also introduces the "remedy" step from the apology process (. . . so I can make it right by you, and make sure I don't make the same mistake again . . .) to further calm the angry party.

CHAPTER 9
Remain Engaged

As one reads this book, there is the danger that apology and disclosure will be seen as something that one can deploy in a single face-to-face sitting with the patient and family, and then move on. If only it were that simple. Apology and disclosure are part of a continuum of respectful care for a patient, not a one-time event. The fifth "R" reminds one to *remain engaged* with the patient and his or her family.

One of the biggest fears patients have in the aftermath of an unexpected, severe outcome is that their physician won't be there for them. In short, they fear being *abandoned* by their provider. Plaintiff attorneys hear clients tell them they felt abandoned all the time.

Hickson's research, mentioned in Chapter 1, found that "patients who saw physicians with the highest number of lawsuits were more likely to complain that their physicians would not listen or return telephone calls, were rude, and did not show respect." My own research with more than 200 surgeons completing a standardized personality assessment suggests that *conflict avoidance* is one component of a set of behaviors that are statistically significant predictors of increased claims risk.[1] If one rereads Hickson's findings above, it seems clear that what patients are describing—physicians who don't listen or return calls, are perceived as rude or not showing respect—is not the intentional bad behavior of irascible physicians. What they are experiencing are physicians who avoid conflict and who don't know how to deal with the conflict they inevitably sense after an unexpected outcome. And because they don't know how to deal with the situation, they withdraw . . . they don't listen, they don't return calls . . . which patients and their families interpret as rude and disrespectful . . . *and they feel abandoned.*

I have personally witnessed the fear of abandonment with one of my patients, when she sustained a severe, unexpected outcome after a laparoscopic cholecystectomy (gallbladder removal):

Ms. K. had been having intermittent pain under her right rib cage, going into her back, associated with nausea for about a month, when a rather severe episode landed her in the emergency room. An ultrasound exam diagnosed gallstones, completing the clinical picture. Her pain was persistent and only partially relieved with pain medication. She was admitted to the hospital and scheduled for surgery by another surgeon.

Her surgery was to be the next day, but the admitting surgeon had a scheduling conflict, so asked me to see Ms. K. I reviewed the chart, introduced myself to her, and went over her history again. I explained the surgery, complete with printed diagrams of the liver and gallbladder, and discussed the risks of the procedure, including bleeding, infection, injury to the tubes draining the liver, and death. Ms. K. worked in the medical profession, so was not ignorant of the process and associated risks.

The surgery proceeded unremarkably. I identified all of the important anatomy, and was confident that only the correct structures had been cut and tied off. Her first post-op day was not unusual, and the morning after surgery, she was eating, her pain was under control, and her lab tests were normal. She had a small amount of bile-colored fluid on one dressing, which I interpreted as "normal" as the bile from the gallbladder was spilled during the

CHAPTER 9
Remain Engaged

surgery (not an uncommon occurrence), and I had used a large amount of saline fluid to wash out the spilled bile. Some of this fluid was slowly coming out of the wound immediately after surgery, and I rationalized that this what I was seeing. With her feeling better, and normal lab tests, I was comfortable sending her home.

Three days later, a Friday, she called and said she was still draining the bile-colored fluid out the incision, but "felt OK." I suggested she come to the office so I could see her, but she declined. (I should have insisted!) She called again on Sunday, understandably distraught, still draining, and I told her I would meet her in the emergency room.

As soon as I saw her, I knew something was wrong. I was concerned that I had cut her bile duct in half—the main tube that drains the liver—one of the most dreaded complications in general surgery. She was tearful and anxious, knowing something was wrong. Her mother, a nurse with a master's degree, also knew things weren't right.

I was completely transparent with them, and told them that I was sorry that this had happened, and it wasn't what either of us had expected. I explained that the cause of the bile leak was one of three things: (1) a small tube between the gallbladder and liver itself had been cut and was leaking, (2) the cystic duct that the gallbladder had been attached to was leaking because the clips had come off, or (3) that I had cut her common bile duct. I could see the concern and fear in her eyes.

I laid out the subsequent diagnostic steps I was going to implement, the consultants who would be involved, and the most likely treatment options. Both Ms. K. and her mother seemed somewhat relieved that I had a clear vision of what was next. (This is, of course, *part of responsibility, as discussed in the previous chapter.)*

I left the room and called the gastroenterologist and explained the situation. He agreed with my assessment and plan and said he would come and see the patient. I went back into the room and told Ms. K. that the gastroenterologist was coming. She looked up at me, and tearfully and fearfully said: "But you're not going to leave me, are you?"

It was then I realized how critical it was to make sure she understand I was with her until she was well. I told her, "I'm responsible for your care, and will be completely available to you. I won't be in the hospital 24 hours a day while you are here, but I am only a telephone call away." The fear I had previously seen on her face melted to a tired smile. She was afraid I was stepping aside and letting an unknown consultant assume care.

Four days later, after a stent, skillfully placed by the gastroenterologist, had failed to seal the leak, I took her back to surgery and, with the assistance of one of my surgical partners, found a small hole (2 millimeters) in her cystic duct. The clips I had originally put on the cystic duct were still in place. I closed the hole with a single stitch. She did phenomenally well and went home a few days later.

This true story seared in my mind the importance of remaining fully engaged with the patient and family after a bad outcome, and how important it is to reassure the patient that "you will be there." It highlights the fact that apology and disclosure are an ongoing process, which requires the provider to be visible and fully engaged until it is clear, *from the patient's perspective,* that everything is OK.

Reference

1. Use of a standardized personality assessment in predicting near-term malpractice claims risk of physicians. 2003. Data on file. Michael S. Woods.

CHAPTER 10
The Evidence That *I'm Sorry* Works

Programs That Work: Practical Lessons in Disclosure and Apology

The telltale sign of a new concept taking hold—and perhaps becoming an emerging trend—is when several large organizations develop practices based on it. I believe this is especially true in industries with a reputation for conservatism, which includes both the health care and insurance industries. Let's look at organizations in these two fields that have implemented full disclosure policies—and with impressive results.

Veterans Affairs Medical Center

The VA Medical Center in Lexington, Kentucky, once had among the highest malpractice claims totals in the VA hospital system. In 1987, after the center lost two malpractice judgments totaling more than $1.5 million, administrators decided to adopt a more proactive policy in medical cases that had the potential to result in litigation. The core concept of the new policy was to maintain a humanistic, care-giving attitude with those who had been harmed, rather than to respond in a defensive and adversarial manner.

As the policy was implemented and ethical issues regarding disclosure arose, the risk management committee had some tough decisions to make. Ultimately, committee members decided the hospital had an obligation to reveal all the details of its investigations to patients and family members affected by errors or negligence, even if they otherwise would not have known that a mishap had occurred.

Basically, this is how the system works: All workers are expected to report both errors and near misses to the hospital risk management committee. When the committee receives a report, members act quickly to determine the root cause. If a patient was harmed by the mistake, the committee generates recommendations for offering aid—such as further medical treatment, assistance in filing for disability benefits, and financial compensation. At a face-to-face meeting, representatives of the hospital apologize to the patient (or family members), emphasize the organization's regret, and explain what corrective actions will take place in response. The chief-of-staff answers medical questions, and the facility's attorney offers a fair settlement.

This approach has helped to defuse anger and negate the desire for revenge, which is so often the patient's motivation for litigation. It's also reduced the VA's legal fees. Patients and/or their attorneys tend to review the clinical information volunteered in good faith by the hospital and are usually willing to negotiate a settlement on the basis of calculable financial losses rather than on the potential for large judgments that might contain punitive damages. The VA's data suggest that apology and good faith go a long way toward mitigating losses. In fact, this policy of disclosure has been so successful and has so greatly benefited the hospital financially that it has been adopted by the entire system of VA hospitals. In 1999 a retroactive study examining the seven-year period from 1990 through 1996 found that there had been 88 malpractice claims against the VA medical center, but the average payment was only $15,622. In contrast, the National Practitioner Data Bank reports that nationally the mean malpractice payment for 2001 was $270,854.

The authors of the VA study acknowledged that barriers exist to adopting similar approaches at nongovernmental hospitals and that private malpractice insurers, who are interested in paying as little as possible, might be inclined to resist such a strategy. However, the University of Michigan Health System and COPIC Companies, a medical malpractice insurance group, adopted a similar approach and achieved results that exceeded expectations.

University of Michigan Health System
The University of Michigan Health System adopted a new policy for handling medical malpractice claims in July 2001.[1] The impetus was to save on defense costs, but what ensued was a program that enhanced patient safety and provider-patient communication.

The policy is based on the following three core principles:

1. Compensating patients quickly and fairly when unreasonable medical care caused a bad outcome
2. Rigorous defense of the staff and hospital when care met the standards or when it is clear that care did not cause an injury
3. A focus on learning from the mistakes made and patient experiences

Simultaneously, the system's legal group began educating the plaintiff's bar and courts about their new approach. The plaintiff's bar enthusiastically supported the effort. Enhanced communication between the groups increased understanding.

Dramatic success was realized in the first year. The university had seven cases go to trial, five of which had the potential to lose many millions of dollars. They won all but one case, which was ultimately settled for $150,000—only a third of what had been demanded. In this year, even after accounting for defense costs, the health system saved $2.2 million. Not bad.

Since then, fewer cases have gone to trial. Claims have been cut by more than half. The plaintiff's bar learned that the university could be approached with honesty and directness, and they would be treated with dignity. If they feel they have a good case, they present all the details to the university, enabling the process to move forward quickly. If they feel they have a marginal case, it is the university's impression that they don't bother, as they know they will be met with a vigorous, aggressive defense, with the best attorneys and best experts. The honesty dividend is paying interest.

Boothman, despite his suggestion that management drives the success of such programs (*see* Chapter 5), has written:

> *My own approach evolved after watching those reactions [of patients who have been dealt with fairly and respectfully, and with open communication], and I became bolder in reassuring our staff that if they would only concentrate on better patient communication and safer patient care, the claims would take care of themselves.*

Boothman has appreciated through this experience that risk management benefits naturally ensure a quality provider-patient relationship.

COPIC Insurance Company

COPIC, a Denver-based medical malpractice insurance company, noted a basic recurring pattern in medical malpractice cases over a 30-year period. The sequence looked something like this:

1. The patient suffered a serious, unexpected outcome.
2. The patient was shocked by the failure to meet his or her expectations.
3. The physician adopted a deny-and-defend attitude toward his or her role in the outcome.
4. When the physician failed to assume accountability for the patient's concerns and needs, the patient became angry.
5. The patient called an attorney and filed a lawsuit.

This pattern led COPIC to develop what the company calls the "3 R's Program"—a plan to resolve medical errors before a malpractice lawsuit resulted. The 3 R's consist of the following:

- Recognizing that the patient has been harmed
- Responding as quickly as possible after the event
- Resolving the patient's medical issues and personal needs

COPIC-insured physicians who participate in the "3Rs Program" agree to call COPIC within 72 hours of making an error or encountering an unanticipated outcome. COPIC specialists then help the physician coordinate a face-to-face meeting with the patient to discuss what went wrong, why it went wrong, and what to expect in the near and long term. Until the medical issues have been resolved, COPIC pays the patient's out-of-pocket expenses plus $100 per day and helps arrange for things such as plane tickets for family members who need to be with their loved one. The program will pay up to $25,000 for out-of-pocket expenses incurred due to the outcome, and $5,000 for lost time.

Of 2,174 cases that met the 3 R's criteria between October 2000 and December 2005, 1,622 cases (75%) did not require *any* payment. Five hundred cases have been closed with some payment, ranging from $95 to the full $30,000. The average payment was $5,680 per case. When this figure is compared to COPIC's claims costs of between $74,643 to $88,056 during the same time period, it becomes clear that an accountant and attorney are not needed to advise an organization what path it should choose. Only 52 cases (2%) have become a legal claim. If one makes the conservative assumption that 15% of the cases in the 3R's program would have become a claim (326) had the 3R's program not existed, the total cost savings is more than $20 million at the low end of the claims costs.

The success rate of the 3 R's program far exceeded the company's expectations. I believe the main reason the program works is that it promotes honest and open communication, including what is, in essence, an apology along with a statement of transparency. It seems doubtful the program would be nearly so successful at avoiding lawsuits if money were offered without the physician's apology and explanation.

While the VA, Michigan, and COPIC programs are viewed favorably because of their results and what they have taught about the power of disclosure, they are based upon, in essence, choreographed communication. The primary focus of these programs is risk management, not apology for apology's sake. I believe that spontaneous, authentic apology, offered as a genuine attempt to heal the physician-patient relationship, accompanied by disclosure, would be even more effective. The major risk advantage of any of these programs—as well as cost savings—occurs because cases that could become claims don't. And the reason they don't is because of the relationship, based on communication. At any rate, these three groundbreaking programs provide overwhelming results that debunk the myth that apology and disclosure contribute to litigation.

Responding to Critics: Overcoming the Cultural and Legal Obstacles to Apology

A big part of the educational effort for proponents of apology and disclosure programs is overcoming the supposed cultural and legal barriers to full disclosure. There is much fear of apology and disclosure in the medical, insurance, and legal communities, but these are emotional, knee-jerk responses that do not hold water. Here are some of the most common challenges posed to apology proponents, and responses that may be used in these discussions.*

Challenge: Doctors will become sitting ducks if they apologize. They'll get their pants sued off.

Response: The current system of deny and defend makes doctors sitting ducks. Doctors and hospital administrators are left to wonder if a process server bringing bad news will follow an unanticipated outcome. That's no way to live. If a mistake occurs, doctors have to ask themselves one question: Would it be better to handle this situation on my terms, or have it fought out by high-priced attorneys in front of a jury of strangers? *Healing Words* provides the protocol to constructively and positively handle errors and bad outcomes.

Challenge: What if *I'm sorry* doesn't work? A doctor has just admitted guilt.

Response: A doctor apologizes for an error and offers compensation, but the compensation is rejected and a lawsuit is initiated. So, the doctor will go to court looking like the person who tried to do the right thing by apologizing and making a fair offer, but was rebuffed. The doctor will be the sympathetic defendant

---

* See "The Sorry Works! Coalition: Making the Case for Full Disclosure" by Doug Wojcieszak, John Banja, and Carole Houk in the *Joint Commission Journal on Quality and Patient Safety,* June 2006. 32(6):344–350.

and the plaintiff will look greedy, which is not the formula for success in the courtroom if you're a trial lawyer. Finally, many states have (or are planning to implement) so-called apology laws whereby an apology from a doctor is not admissible in court.

<u>Challenge:</u> Lawyers simply file too many lawsuits in my hometown for the *Healing Words* approach to be successful.

<u>Response:</u> If a region or county is considered to be friendly to plaintiffs' attorneys, all the more reason for doctors to implement apology and disclosure. Doctors, hospital administrators, and insurers should do everything possible to make sure that patients and families don't leave their offices angry in litigious regions. A good apology and disclosure program provides the protocol and methods to alleviate anger and significantly diminish the chances of lawsuits being filed, especially in the most litigious areas. An overly aggressive trial attorney is powerless without an angry plaintiff.

<u>Challenge:</u> But not all bad medical outcomes are the result of errors. Sometimes people just die or are injured despite the best efforts of a medical staff. We can't be handing out checks every time someone dies or doesn't heal completely.

<u>Response:</u> People die from medical errors, but not all deaths are caused by medical errors. Many times the standard of care is met, but people still die or do not completely heal. Doctors and hospitals certainly should not be expected to "hand out checks" under these circumstances. However, they still need to communicate with patients and families. This lack of communication and a perception of a cover-up cause lawsuits even when the standard of care is met.

Hospitals that practice apology develop a reputation for honesty with local plaintiffs' attorneys. If the hospital plans to contest a case (no apology or settlement), local attorneys learn that such cases are probably without merit and not worth pursuing. As mentioned earlier, this effect is called "the honesty dividend."

Challenge: Kraman developed apology in a VA hospital. \It will never work in a private hospital.

Response: Kaiser Hospitals and Catholic Healthcare West show this to be untrue. Furthermore, as more and more hospitals become captive insurers, apology and disclosure will become easier to implement. Insurance companies are also starting to seriously study apology, and the story of Dr. Frederick van Pelt shows how individual practitioners can implement apology and disclosure, even without approval from their insurer. Perhaps doing the right thing is the way to go!

Dr. van Pelt's Story

When a medical mishap turned Linda Kenney's routine ankle surgery into a chilling brush with death, the family quickly paid a visit to a lawyer's office. The jury, the family suspected, would likely show little mercy to the anesthesiologist, Frederick van Pelt, who inadvertently injected a painkilling drug in the wrong place, causing Ms. Kenney's heart to stop. To restart it, doctors at the Brigham and Women's hospital sliced her chest and cracked open her rib cage. Ms. Kenney's husband, Kevin, "wanted to kill the anesthesiologist, flatten him," says the 41-year-old mother of three.

But then, Dr. van Pelt broke with convention. Against the hospital's advice, he wrote Ms. Kenney a personal letter saying he was "deeply saddened" by her suffering. Later, over coffee at a suburban diner, he apologized for the terrible accident.

"I found out he was a real person," Ms. Kenney says. "He made an effort to seek me out and say he was sorry I suffered." Moved by the doctor's contrition, Ms. Kenney dropped her plans to sue.

Source: *Wall Street Journal*, May 18, 2004.

Challenge: Apology and disclosure increase settlements, which means more doctors get reported to the disciplinary board.

Response: Not necessarily. According to the *National Practitioner Database Guidebook*, "a payment made as a result of a suit or claim solely against an entity that does not identify an individual practitioner is not reportable." The *Guidebook* also says, "medical malpractice payments are limited to exchanges of money and must be the result of a written complaint or claim demanding monetary payment for damages." This suggests if disclosure is rigorous, forthright, and speedy, then a written claim/complaint may be avoided and, thus, physicians' names not reported.

The Greatest Hurdles of All . . .

Medical culture and physician behavior. John Banja, a bioethics professor, notes in *Medical Errors and Medical Narcissism*:

> *Expressions of professional narcissism, hyperdefensiveness, and blame shifting are coping mechanisms that help health care professionals manage the dissonance between their perfectionist aspirations and the reality of their imperfect selves and environments. Consider, though, how the psychological pain deriving from error realization can be compounded by the professional's feeling obligated to disclose the error and apologize for it. Apologizing for errors requires that the professional give up the pretensions, beliefs, and posturing that accompany the conviction that he or she must be perfect . . . disclosure and apology following a serious error might be psychologically impossible.*

CHAPTER 10
The Evidence That *I'm Sorry* Works

Cultural change will be difficult, but the benefits of apology and disclosure certainly merit the effort.

Reference
1. Boothman, R.: Apologies and a strong defense at the University of Michigan Health System. *The Physician Executive* pp. 7–10, Mar.–Apr. 2006.

CHAPTER 11
The Ethical Debate About Disclosure

*Often, the less there is to justify a traditional custom,
the harder it is to get rid of it.*
                                        —Mark Twain

Can apology alone salvage the relationship between a doctor and a patient who has experienced an unexpected outcome? As we have seen, patients also want to know—and have a right to know—the details of what went awry when a medical intervention leaves them sicker than they were before treatment.

In medicine, reconstructing the events leading up to an adverse outcome is a process commonly called *disclosure.* Unfortunately, that term has negative connotations in society at large, where it's used to describe the revelation of sordid—or at least unflattering—personal information. For this reason, I prefer to use the phrase *statement of transparency,* which reflects honesty, openness, and a proactive willingness to share information with patients—including details that may not shine a flattering light on the health care provider. From this point on, when you see the phrase *statement of transparency,* keep in mind that I'm referring to disclosure.

> *I prefer to use the phrase* statement of transparency, *which reflects honesty, openness, and a proactive willingness to share information with patients*

There are three major reasons that making a statement of transparency is important. First of all, it's the right thing to do ethically. Second, the medical profession is being mandated to inform patients about the details of adverse events. Finally, the profession and their organizations will benefit from the honesty dividend.

The Patient Perspective on Disclosure

Research shows that patients want to know about bad outcomes and medical errors, even those that don't cause serious or lasting harm. Interestingly, but not surprisingly, Gallagher found that while patients identify "truthfulness" and "compassion" as having primary importance in the disclosure process, physicians say "truthfulness" and "objectivity" are the qualities that matter most. Gallagher's focus groups revealed that patients overwhelmingly want to know the following:

- What happened?
- How will this affect my health in the short term? In the long term?
- Why did this happen?
- What is being done to treat the problem I have now?
- Who will bear the cost of this error or complication?
- What will you do to protect other patients from a similar mistake?

Gallagher's findings are supported by research conducted by Leonard J. Marcus, director of the Harvard School of Public Health's Program for Healthcare Negotiation and Conflict Resolution. Marcus analyzed transcripts of mediation sessions to determine what patients really want, and he discovered three main requirements: an explanation of what happened, an apology, and assurances that changes would be made to protect other patients from the same kind of harm.

Conspicuously absent from both lists is the desire to know who caused the problem.

Gallagher's focus groups revealed that patients want the doctor to take the initiative to explain situations to them. They don't want to have to interrogate the physician to get the whole story. While many physicians are wary of revealing information due to concerns about litigation, patients seek explanations not to affix blame, but simply because they want to understand. After all, their health is in jeopardy.

Note that not a single doctor in Gallagher's focus groups said he or she would offer a patient, in the aftermath of an error, an explanation about steps that would be taken to prevent similar mistakes in the future. Yet this is something patients have indicated they want to hear. And I can understand why! Not only does talking about the prevention of future slip-ups put the discussion in a more positive light, it allows people who've had these experiences to make sense of them—to take comfort in knowing that others may benefit from their distress. If there is a silver lining to the dark cloud of medical errors, it's that they can expose flawed policies and procedures, serving as a catalyst to make health care safer.

The Code of Medical Ethics Demands Disclosure

Ethics, compassion, caring, concern, and the avid pursuit of always doing right by patients theoretically drive the profession of medicine. Yet many physicians may not know what medical organizations have to say about honesty in communicating errors or complications to patients. The American Medical Association (AMA) has had a Code of Medical Ethics for some time. Section 8.12 states:

It is a fundamental ethical requirement that a physician should at all times deal honestly and openly with patients. Patients have a right to know their past and present medical status and to be free of any mistaken beliefs concerning their conditions. Situations occasionally occur in which a patient suffers significant medical complications that may have resulted from the physician's mistake or judgment. In these situations, the physician is ethically required to inform the patient of all the facts necessary to ensure understanding of what has occurred. Only through full disclosure is a patient able to make informed decisions regarding future medical care.

Concern regarding legal liability that might result following truthful disclosure should not affect the physician's honesty with a patient.

Please note this specific phrase: *The physician is ethically required to inform the patient of all the facts necessary to ensure understanding of what has occurred.* If a patient has an unexpected outcome, he or she has the right to know what happened, why it happened (to the extent known), and what is being done to rectify the situation. I don't believe physicians expect anything less when members of their families suffer complications.

Also note the last sentence of the AMA's code: *Concern regarding legal liability that might result following truthful disclosure should not affect the physician's honesty with a patient.* This statement presents an interesting conundrum for physicians because some medical malpractice insurers will cancel their policies for providing full disclosure if a case ultimately lands in court. This highlights yet another situation in medicine in which there is a misalignment between what people want from physicians and what they get. The good news, of course, is that evidence suggests a malpractice claim is less likely to be filed if a physician has provided a statement of transparency as part of an apology.

The Joint Commission on Accreditation of Healthcare Organizations, the premier accrediting body for health care in the United States, also requires that hospitals inform patients and, when appropriate, their families about unanticipated outcomes of care, treatment, and services. In the "Ethics, Rights, and Responsibilities" chapter in the *2006 Comprehensive Accreditation Manual for Hospitals*, Standard RI.2.90 states: "Patients and, when appropriate, their families are informed about the outcomes of care, treatment, and service that have been provided, including unanticipated outcomes." It goes on to specify that "the responsible licensed independent practitioner or his or her designee informs the patient . . . about those unanticipated outcomes . . . when the patient is not already aware of the occurrence, or further discussion is needed." Again, the responsibility is clearly with the health care provider to honestly communicate with the patient.

Disclosure Is Ongoing Informed Consent

Informed consent is the process by which fully informed patients participate in decisions regarding their medical care. It stems from a patient's legal and ethical right to choose what happens to his or her body, and it should be characterized by mutual respect and shared decision making. Informed consent is the vehicle by which patients express their personal treatment preferences and maintain their autonomy. Informed consent should include the following:

• A detailed explanation of the treatment, procedure, or

decision in question
- Options for alternative treatments
- The benefits, risks, and uncertainties surrounding each treatment option

Ideally, the patient would understand the options given, assess each one, and select the preferred option before initiating treatment.

As I noted earlier, lawsuits result from unmet patient expectations. The consent process is the time for physicians to have frank, clearly articulated conversations with patients regarding their expectations as well as potential risks and complications. If a patient has expectations the physician considers unrealistic, those should be clarified before proceeding.

The legal standard of informed consent has varied through the years, as follows:

The past: The legal standard applied to informed consent in the past mandated that the information given was what a reasonable and prudent physician would tell a patient. This, obviously, gave more weight to what the physician thought was important than what the patient might want to know. This standard was not designed to empower patients and did not respect their autonomy.

The present: The present legal standard for informed consent states that the information provided should be what reasonable patients need to know to make a rational decision. This is a more patient-centered, respectful approach that strives to preserve patient autonomy. The phrase "need to know," however, still sets a physician-determined limit on what is disclosed to the patient.

The future: The emerging standard for informed consent is the ideal—a patient-specific, subjective standard. This standard requires physicians to ask themselves, *"What information does this specific patient need to know and understand to make a decision?"* It eliminates the concepts of "reasonable" or "average" patients and requires information to be tailored specifically to an individual. It takes into account that different patients may want to hear very different levels of detail, depending on their values, goals, cultural biases, and capability to understand clinical information. This standard obviously requires the greatest amount of skilled communication from the physician.

Obviously, when complications arise or errors occur, a patient's expectations regarding his or her prognosis must necessarily change. Decisions concerning care will have to be revisited—and in those instances, disclosure acts as ongoing informed consent.

Direct analogies can be made between the histories of informed consent standards and disclosure standards. Because we're talking about disclosure as an extension of the consent process, let's take a look at the following:

The past standard of disclosure: Before the litigious environment of the last 20 years, the standard for disclosure might have been described in terms similar to the past standard for consent: what a reasonable and prudent physician would tell a patient. This resulted in the patient receiving only a minimum amount of information. Compounding the problem was the typical patient's unwillingness to confront the physician or request information—that was the era when doctors were gods (well, authority figures at least). Picture a physician patting a patient on the head and saying, "Don't worry—we'll take good care of you," and you have a good idea of just how this past standard played out.

The present standard of disclosure: Too many doctors and hospitals do not even begin to fulfill the ethical consent standard of "what reasonable patients need to know to make a rational decision." Sometimes the health provider's approach is to keep information away from the patient—or to provide only the minimum required to satisfy the patient's questions. This mindset is based on a flawed view of risk management, and it places the physician (or his organization) in an adversarial role with the patients in his or her care. It could be argued that this has been and continues to be a period of little-to-no meaningful disclosure.

The evolving standard of disclosure: The emerging state of disclosure, a "statement of transparency," as mentioned earlier, is both similar to and different from the informed consent processes described above. While the amount of information and detail that individual patients wish to know about an unanticipated outcome or error may vary, one thing is clear: Everyone has the right to hear an apology, to be informed of what can be expected in the near and long-term future, and to be reassured that he or she will not be abandoned.

A Lesson from the Friendly Skies

The Institute of Medicine's (IOM) now infamous report on medical errors estimates that as many as 98,000 people die in hospitals each year due to medical errors. Consequently, the federal government has turned a great deal of attention to patient safety. While the IOM report recommends that the federal government require public disclosure of medical errors, organized medicine has strongly resisted.

One objection is that reporting errors in public forums might lead to sensationalism by the media and unwarranted public mistrust of the health care system. Proponents of mandatory error reporting believe this concern could be mitigated by keeping sensitive information from the public. They're in favor of doing away with the current culture of blame by instituting a nonpunitive, confidential system in which errors would be disclosed to authorities who would use the data in a proactive way.

The IOM's reason for recommending mandatory disclosure makes good sense. Medical errors can nearly always be traced back to a breakdown of systems as opposed to an individual human error. Health care is a complex arrangement of interdependent parts that provide multiple checkpoints for catching errors. For example, a pharmacist alerts a doctor that his prescribed dose is too high for a child.

But this system also provides multiple points where breakdowns can occur—for instance, a doctor is forced to make a diagnosis without reviewing past notes because a patient's chart was misfiled. Disclosing errors instead of covering them up can pinpoint and fix weak links in the system, resulting in fewer errors down the line.

The airline industry offers a compelling model of success. Airlines cannot cover up their mistakes—plane crashes are highly visible events. Yet the industry not only survives such catastrophes, it actually bolsters public confidence by revealing the details of its investigations and the resulting efforts to prevent similar mishaps. Therefore, the traveling public believes the airlines are committed to safety and has confidence that the dangers of air travel are minimal. The statistics support this: In 1976 the risk of dying in an airplane accident was one in two million.

Today—despite a huge increase in the number of flights and passengers per day—the risk is one in eight million, a fourfold increase in safety.

The Aviation Safety Reporting System (ASRS), a nonpunitive error reporting system administered by NASA for the Federal Aviation Administration, has contributed greatly to safety improvements in the industry. Any airline employee who makes an error or witnesses a near miss must fill out an incident report. That person's identity is removed from the report before anyone at the airline sees it, and systems experts then analyze the reports to gain insights that are incorporated into future training programs. Thanks to this system, the number of accidents attributed to both human error and system breakdowns has plummeted.

Many physicians are skeptical that a similar system could work in medicine. They fear individuals who make medical errors would be singled out and somehow punished, despite the fact that the ASRS has successfully overcome all issues of confidentiality, anonymity, and retaliatory discipline in its own system. And they argue—probably correctly—that physicians would resist being singled out for additional training designed to prevent future errors. (Pilots routinely receive training about new policies and procedures designed to enhance safety when weaknesses in the system are revealed.)

I believe a system comparable to the one employed by commercial aviation would contribute to the development of a similar culture of safety in medicine. Until such time, however, the use of authentic apology and statements of transparency will help rebuild the public confidence that's shaken when errors occur.

The Honesty Dividend

One of the major, often unappreciated benefits of apology and disclosure in health care is the *honesty dividend*. It is a simple concept, really, with two distinct benefits to providers and their organizations.

When a physician or organization becomes known for dealing with patients and their families with honesty and transparency in *all* circumstances, the public's perception of them (the doctor and the organization) begins to shift. Patients begin to understand that there are no secrets, and that if something bad happens, they will be treated respectfully and provided with a full account of known details surrounding the event. The community served by the hospital begins to give the organization and the doctors who practice there the benefit of the doubt, as they develop the confidence that they will be dealt with fairly, with respect and empathy.

The second component to the honesty dividend is the potential to directly reduce legal expenses. An apology and disclosure program helps physicians and their organizations develop or restore a reputation for being straight shooters when they refuse to settle a malpractice claim brought against them. Also, trial lawyers quickly learn that the bad outcome does not likely involve negligence and is not worth pursuing. Pursuit of litigation will be, more often than not, a financial sinkhole for plaintiffs and their attorneys. Promoting transparency takes the guesswork out of medical malpractice lawsuits and allows patients and lawyers to clearly see which cases have merit and in which cases there is real fault. Apology and disclosure, and, when appropriate, offering fair compensation for any identified errors, dissipate anger, which, as we have learned, is the driver of medical malpractice lawsuits.

Apology, Liability, and the Law

While it is not yet a trend, legislators are beginning to remove some of the stumbling blocks to apology. At the end of the last decade, both legal academicians and policy makers began to raise the following question: Should apologies be admissible evidence as proof of fault in civil cases?

Apology laws—those that deny the admissibility of an apology to support a claim—have been around for some time. In the 1970s, the daughter of a Massachusetts state senator was struck and killed by a car. The father was angry that the driver never expressed any remorse, but soon learned that under then-existing evidence laws, the driver dared not apologize because it could have constituted an admission of fault. Years later, the senator sponsored a bill that ultimately came to exclude "expressions of sympathy and benevolence" made after an accident to prove liability in a civil suit.

Benevolent gestures are defined as actions that convey a sense of compassion or commiseration. Examples include verbal expressions of apology or regret; written messages, including sympathy cards; and respectful conduct, such as sending flowers or attending a funeral or memorial service.

Texas passed a similar law in 1999 and California in 2000. A handful of other states followed. These laws were not specific to medical errors but to accidents in general. As written, however, slight differences in the phrasing of an apology could have a profoundly different effect on litigation. Certain kinds of apologies are protected and others are not. Saying *I'm sorry you were hurt*, for example, carries completely different legal ramifications than saying *I'm sorry I hurt you*.

CHAPTER 11
The Ethical Debate About Disclosure

Today there is ongoing debate among legal scholars and policy makers as to whether all sorts of apologies—including those that hint at personal fault—should become inadmissible evidence in civil lawsuits. In 2003 Colorado became the first state to pass a law specific to medical apology, making statements of contrition by doctors inadmissible to support claims of physician liability. I believe other states will follow, and I hope that risk management with a humanistic approach will someday become the norm.

Reference
1. Doug Wojcieszak, from the SorryWorks! Web site.
   http://www.sorryworks.net/media17.phtml (accessed Jun. 7, 2006).

CHAPTER 12
Building a Culture of Civility

Creating the Culture You Want

The beautiful thing about apology and disclosure is that it can be implemented today. In my opinion, providers really don't need permission from anyone. Your organization doesn't need to involve the state legislators. You don't have to call the governor. We don't need Hillary Clinton (although we would welcome her help). As Nike has told us for years: Just Do It.

Building a culture of apology doesn't begin with a focus on patients. It doesn't begin with a focus on employees. It begins by focusing on *your own behaviors and communication style* and paying attention to the basic concepts of civility. If you desire an organization where apology is offered when normal social circumstances would expect as much, then civility must be infused into the culture.

Ask yourself the following questions:

- Do you routinely say "Hello" and smile to everyone you meet in your organization, acknowledging their presence?
- Do you routinely say "excuse me" when you interrupt a fellow provider, patient, or family member?
- Do you routinely say "thank you" to coworkers, for even small things that they are expected to do?
- Do you, as a surgeon, routinely say "thank you" for the assistance the scrub nurse and assistants give you?
- Do you listen—*really listen*—to what others say to you? Or do you disregard what is said and proceed however you want?

- Do you show everyone the same respect and consideration, regardless of their position or title?

If you answered "yes" to each of these things, you are acting with civility. If not, perhaps you need to evaluate whether you are showing your best side.

Apology is just one behavior of a civil environment, but a crucial one. As you have learned, apology is about respect, trust, humility, and valuing the relationship. Who would deny that these are important components of our relationships in health care, whether with our fellow providers, patients, or patient families?

To change the culture of an organization, it takes only one committed person, forming an epicenter for change. If that person makes a commitment to become more aware of the small violations for which an apology may be offered, he or she sets a visible example. Soon, like-minded, civilly acting individuals will begin to do the same. And slowly, imperceptibly at first, the organization's culture will shift.

Why would one want to build a culture of civility, beginning with the simple concept of apology? Patients are passive (sometimes active) observers of the organization's environment. While we speak of organizational behavior, there is really only the behavior of individuals within the organization. The organization's tone is determined by the collective behavior displayed by the employees and providers. When patients see physicians apologize to nurses and other providers on the health care team as a matter of civil behavior and when patients see nurses apologize to physicians and other coworkers, and so on, it establishes the provider's and organization's credibility In the event of a medical error or a bad outcome, when a provider apologizes to the patient and family, it has credibility—it is believable—because they have witnessed an entire organization acting with civility, of which one of the most visible manifestations is respectful and considerate apology.

Civility: The Hope for Health Care

Of course, civility should go beyond our work as health care providers. Just about the most important thing we do in life is interact with other human beings: spouse, children, parents, friends, coworkers . . . and in health care, patients. As P. M. Forni, the cofounder of the Civility Initiative at Johns Hopkins, puts it, "A crucial measure of our success in life is the way we treat one another every day of our lives."

In health care, we interact with patients who feel vulnerable and afraid. The relationship skills of health care providers determine the *quality* of the health care experience for all involved, whether patient, nurse, aide, physician, or pharmacist.

As medicine understands more and more about the human body and its ailments, and uses ever-increasingly complex and elegant technology to treat patients, it seems we drift further away from humanism and the very real needs of the people we treat.

For the better part of a decade, I have promoted physician leadership as the key to health care's ills—plummeting patient satisfaction, malpractice spiraling out of control, patient safety violations, and health care practitioners who discourage young people from entering a profession that can be rewarding in ways others cannot. I now believe the key is more basic, and understandable, than leadership. The key is civility . . . from and between providers,[1] patients, administrators, and even attorneys.

Civility is a code of behavior based on respect, restraint, and responsibility. There are six principles of civility:

1. Respect
2. Empathy
3. Flexibility
4. Interest in other cultures
5. Tolerance
6. Technical skills

These principles are critical to catapulting us over the hurdles we face in health care, leaving them far behind in the mist of the past. To understanding them, you need only to be a human being. You don't need an M.D., R.N., or any other degree. Committing to the principles allows health care providers to be more effective in what they strive to do in the first place—care for others.

Civility First

According to P. M. Forni, from whom I draw on for much of the work in this chapter, civility is a code of behavior based on respect, restraint, and responsibility. There are three ways to interpret civility, or civil behavior[1]:

1. Ethically neutral: Acting with civility is socially expedient; it lubricates our social interactions. By acting with civility, others like to be with us.
2. Ethically: Acting with civility gives us a benevolent awareness of others and that our behaviors affect those around us. Civility helps us distinguish between right and wrong, especially with regard to how we treat others.

3. Aesthetics: Acting with civility is considered refined and sophisticated and is used to please others. This is illustrated by the Italian term *sprezzatura*, loosely translated as "the art of doing things gracefully."

We don't have to choose between the various interpretations, because all are valid and worthwhile reasons to behave with civility.

Why Civility? Why Now?

At first blush, the need for civility may seem obscure. Closer examination, however, leads one to a conclusion that civility is the key to transforming health care. Common knowledge does not imply common practice. We all have equilibrium. We all have balance, but that doesn't mean one who has never been on a bike can simply get on and pedal off. We all have the *ability* to float in water, but we must *learn* to swim. To use a computer analogy, we all are made with hardware to run the civility "program," but may have loaded the wrong software (that is, learned and accepted less-than-civil behavior from ourselves and others).[1] Physicians particularly may run the wrong software, "downloaded" during training; so much of our behavior is learned.

There are clear social and personal benefits to acting with civility:

1. Civility is connected to the principle of respect for other people. A civil individual treats all others as ends in themselves, as intrinsically valuable individuals, rather than to serve some immediate need or desire. The latter form of treatment is, in essence, slavery. In health care, a common observation is seeing physicians treat nurses and other providers as "tools of patient care" instead of valued team

members. Such treatment is disrespectful and counter to the team-based care approach that has been demonstrated to be superior to more traditional care. Further, it has been demonstrated that nurses treat other employees poorly at the same rate as physicians, implying that, if behavior goes uncorrected, it spawns a culture of incivility in the organization.[2]

2. There is a connection between incivility, business results, and violence. In the everyday workplace, acts of disrespect are spiraling out of control. More than 45% of respondents in a survey of 800 people, conducted by the University of North Carolina at Chapel Hill's Kenan-Flagler Business School, contemplated changing jobs because of rudeness, and 12% actually changed jobs.[3] A good number of violent incidents have been linked to incivility in the workplace. What's this got to do with health care? Thirty percent of 1,200 individuals interviewed knew of a nurse who quit his or her job due to the behavior of a physician.[4] The cost to organizations in turnover costs is horrific, estimated in 1997 dollars to be $150,000 per disruptive physician.[5] (Imagine what this would be if adjusted for inflation!) Further, it is my belief, supported by data, that physician violations of the principles of civility are *the* major generators of medical malpractice claims. Multiple "small violations" across time by a physician—habitually being late in the clinic, telling patients that he or she will "call with the lab results" and failing to do so, interrupting, limiting questions or controlling the conversation during the office visit, and failing to apologize for the various civility violations (much less for unexpected outcomes or errors)—create conditions that lead patients to sue when an outcome is less than expected. Patients are angry at the physician before

the infraction that leads them to sue. Civility matters!

3. There is a connection between civility and personal well-being. Many high-quality studies have clearly documented that civility is not just good form, but a matter of good health. We find purpose and meaning in our relationships. Consider these findings[6]:

Serious diseases in men who are not close to their parents occur at a rate of 100%. Men with warm relationships with their parents report only a 47% rate of similar illness.

People living in isolation die at a rate of 1.9 to 3.1 times higher than those who are well integrated in their social environment. People who are part of diverse social networks are more effective at fighting off viral illness. The immune systems of couples who argue a lot are weaker than those of couples who don't. The quality of our lives depends on the quality of our relationships with others, but the quality of our relationships depends upon our relational skills. The six principles of civility serve as our guide for how to behave toward our fellow humans. Each principle can be learned and cultivated, if one is open to self-examination, feedback, and personal improvement.

References
1. Forni, P. M.: Lecture. International Association of Protocol Consultants Conference, Washington, DC, May 4–6, 2006.
2. *Am J Nurs.* 105(1):54–64. 2005
3. Etiquette crisis at work. *CNN Money,* Nov. 29, 1999.
4. Rosenstein A.: *AJN,* 102: Jun. 2002.
5. Pfifferling J.: Managing the unmanageable: The disruptive physician. *Family Practice Management* Nov.–Dec. 1997.
6. Forni P. M.: *Choosing Civility. The Twenty-five Rules of Considerate Conduct.* New York: St. Martin's Press, 2002, pp. 28–30.

CHAPTER 13
Boot Camp for Authentic Relationships

Patients might not be able to quickly gauge whether a physician is competent in his or her specialty, but they know almost immediately whether they're inclined to like him or her. This is important, because the nature of the doctor-patient relationship affects the quality of health care, and the initial interaction between a doctor and patient can set the tone for their relationship.

Sincerity—or the seeming lack of it—is one of the first qualities a patient is likely to sense in a doctor. Sincerity shows in a physician's genuine, authentic attempts to see, listen to, speak to, understand, and connect with the patient. *Authentic* here means conveying a genuine interest in and respect for the person. This is something that cannot be faked by using a communication technique learned as a way to avoid lawsuits.

Authentic communication includes the kind of informational transparency that I discussed earlier, but it is much more than that. It is bidirectional interaction between two people that begins the moment eyes meet and evolves into a complex, multidimensional experience. Authentic communication involves not only speech, but much subtler cues, including body language. While much of the responsibility for clear communication falls to the physician, it is a two-way street.

Seeing Authentically

To establish effective communication, physicians must understand the context of the patient's situation—not only medically, but socially and culturally as well. When first meeting patients,

> *Considering that one in every five patients walking into a doctor's office has poor health literacy, it only makes sense for physicians to pay attention to these clues.*

physicians should look for visual signs of their lifestyles: How is the patient dressed? Does he or she look you in the eye? What about hygiene? Is he or she visibly in pain or fearful? Such observations can help a physician determine a patient's health choices and health literacy—the ability to express and formulate questions as well as to understand clinical explanations. Considering that one in every five patients walking into a doctor's office has poor health literacy, it only makes sense for physicians to pay attention to these clues.

This is terribly important because the evolving standard of informed consent requires physicians to tailor the information dispensed to the individual patient's needs. And the patient's ability to understand and follow instructions will determine how faithfully he or she complies with the prescribed treatment plan, affecting both outcome and safety. In one study of pediatric patients, 35% of adverse outcomes were attributed at least partially to communication failures between clinicians or between clinician and parents.[1]

Patients formulate their first impressions of a doctor through visual perceptions. As consumers contracting for a service, they are very likely to notice whether the provider seems respectful. A physician who neglects to maintain eye contact and stares at the patient's chart or takes notes incessantly throughout the visit comes across as closed off to the patient. Patients want and deserve the full attention of their doctors, and they may understandably grow resentful and dissatisfied when they don't get it. They may also feel distrustful toward a physician who appears fatigued, disheveled, or distracted.

Speaking Authentically

Arguably the most important component of patient-physician communication is speech. Few things will derail the physician-patient relationship more surely than an introduction consisting of a half-hearted, limp handshake accompanied by a cheerless *"Hello, I'm Dr. So-and-So"* that sounds like a voice-mail recording.

I personally believe that physicians should introduce themselves by first name. I encourage patients to call me "Mike," not "Dr. Woods." Many doctors disagree with me on this, but I know from conversations with patients that it helps put them at ease. It levels the playing field, putting doctor and patient on the same plane. Insisting on using a title constructs a barrier to open, authentic dialogue. Physician-researcher Howard Waitzkin, M.D., found that doctors often maintain a style of "high control" when communicating with patients. Elevating themselves with titles is part of this manipulation. Frankly, the days when patients held physicians in reverence and awe are gone.

Many physicians use intimidating question-and-answer techniques to maintain control—although they may not be aware that's what they're doing. Most office visits begin with an exchange of information. But often, physician-initiated questions come in machine-gun fashion and focus only on the main complaint. Few pauses are provided for the patient to respond fully. One study demonstrated that physicians on average give patients only 22 seconds to answer a question before cutting them off.

It is not uncommon these days for physicians to rely on interview notes taken by nurses as a substitute for personally hearing the patient out. As health care becomes increasingly consumer-driven and the World Wide Web makes medical information even more easily accessible, patients will have more questions than ever before and expect their doctors to discuss their conditions with them in detail, without having nurses or office staff act as intermediaries. Doctors should offer this without waiting for their patients to request it.

It is absolutely critical to patient care, compliance, and safety that physicians respond to patients at their level of understanding. Never dispense a prescription without first ascertaining that the patient knows what it's for. A patient given medication for hypertension needs to know that hypertension means high blood pressure, which carries an increased risk of heart attack. Don't assume that the patient knows this just because everyone in your acquaintance does.

On the other hand, patients with above-average intelligence or high health literacy don't appreciate being "talked down to." Waitzkin, in his study on doctor-patient communication, noted that doctors tend to underestimate the patient's desire for information. Those who have the ability to understand clinical explanations often want to hear an exact diagnosis—so offer to write down the medical terms that describe their illness, symptoms, or diagnostic tests that will be used. Physicians who insist on using either tech-talk or baby-talk with patients are, frankly, attempting to maintain a controlling position. While it may take some innovative, on-the-feet thinking to adjust clinical explanations to an individual's specific level of understanding, physicians should make the effort.

CHAPTER 13
Boot Camp for Authentic Relationships

Listening Authentically

Authentic listening requires listening not only with your ears, but also with your heart to comprehend the feelings beneath the words. Kevin Cashman, author of *Leadership from the Inside Out*, says this about authentic listening:

> We hear the words, but do we also "hear" the emotions, fears, underlying concerns? Authentic listening is not a technique. It is centered in compassion and in a concern for the other person that goes beyond our self-centered needs. Listening authentically is centered in the principle of psychological reciprocity: To influence others, we must first be open to their influence.

I suspect many physicians are guilty of listening selectively for only the bits of information they deem "useful" in formulating a diagnosis. Instead, they should listen with intensity, as if it were the first time they'd ever heard such a story. This holds true even if the patient has told the same story over and over again.

Authentic listening—being able to "hear" the emotions, fears, and underlying concerns, as Cashman puts it—is even more important in a medical setting in which a patient experiences an unexpected outcome or complication. The patient's predominant emotion may be fear, but physicians may miss this if it isn't expressly verbalized. In other words, the ability to listen authentically requires seeing authentically as well.

Of course, even with the best effort and intentions, the potential for misunderstanding always exists. After all, we interpret what we hear based on our worldview. Differences in cultural heritage, spiritual beliefs, education, and socioeconomic levels between physician and patient can result in varying interpretations and perceptions of the same reality. Physicians need to be sensitive to these incongruent points of view. For example, it's easy to see how a frightened patient could regard a severe allergic reaction to a new drug as a "medical error," when the doctor in fact had no way of predicting the allergy. Hearing the fear and confusion behind the patient's questions or angry accusations can go a long way toward formulating an empathetic response.

Writing Authentically

Whenever and wherever a physician writes about a patient, the notes should be clear, honest, and respectful. Furthermore, the writing should be legible and neat. Just as the physician is accountable for learning to speak with clarity and accuracy, he or she is also accountable for the physical act of writing clearly and accurately. Physicians who fail to write legibly either neglect to understand or refuse to acknowledge that illegible handwriting jeopardizes patient safety.

Handwriting is a learned skill, and with focus and practice everyone can write legibly. In recognition of this, Cedars-Sinai Medical Center in Los Angeles offers a handwriting class to physicians, and Indiana University Medical School has added penmanship to its curriculum. In the end, if a physician cannot write legibly, it is his or her responsibility to choose another method for documentation, such as dictating an entry to the patient's record, even if he or she has to pay for it. The reason for clear written communication is obvious from a patient safety standpoint—both in a patient record that another clinician may have to rely on at some point and on the prescription pad, because many drugs have names that look alike.

Authentic Body Language

Have you ever found yourself trying to speak to someone who

was fidgeting with a pen or a paper clip? Intermittently glancing at the TV? Flipping the pages of a magazine? What kind of non-verbal messages did you receive in these scenarios? You probably felt the other person was pretending to listen but not really hearing you at all.

When you see a patient in the office or the hospital, sit down within touching distance. The patient perceives a standing physician very differently than a physician who is seated. One study asked hospitalized patients to estimate the amount of time their doctors spent with them. All the doctors' visits lasted exactly 5 minutes, yet patients who saw a standing physician estimated the visit lasted about 2 or 3 minutes, while those whose physicians pulled a chair up to the bedside perceived the visit to have lasted 15 minutes. The message of the standing physician is *I'm in a hurry, so let's get this over with!* The message of the physician who sits is *I've got as much time as you need.* While in reality the amount of time spent is the same, the patient's assessment is very different.

Another critical issue of body language is eye contact. Look at your patient. Don't flip through the chart. If you typically make notes in the chart during an appointment, ask the patient if it's okay—yes, ask for permission—or do it after you leave the room. Using periods of eye contact, with appropriate pauses in between, is common social etiquette. Failure to make adequate eye contact engenders mistrust. And whether standing or sitting, don't cross your arms. It sends the message that you are trying to keep a barrier between yourself and the patient, or that you are in a hurry.

Trust Accrual and Trust Equity

Establishing a relationship with another person—any person—

requires that you demonstrate trustworthiness. Once upon a time, merely having an "M.D." behind your name earned trust. Today, from a patient's perspective, the credentials behind the name do not necessarily mean anything but clinical competence—and sometimes even that is no longer assumed.

Trust is established over time. It can be challenging to gain a patient's trust in the all-too-common 10-minute office visit or hospital consult. And trust is difficult to foster when a physician does not consistently see the same patient, when there is no provider-patient continuity. In some practices, it's the norm for whoever is "on" that day to see the patient in the office or hospital. Many OB/GYN groups rotate their pregnant patients through multiple partners because they rotate call. From both a relationship and risk management standpoint, this is an uncertain practice. In the event of a bad outcome, there's an increased likelihood of a malpractice claim, for the simple reason that the patient did not build a trusting relationship with the doctor she feels is responsible.

In today's health care environment, distrust is the norm until a patient has spent sufficient time with a doctor to establish a relationship. One approach to understanding trust is to think about it in banking terms. Trust accrual occurs over a period of time, just as a relationship is built one office visit at a time. An extended first visit is particularly helpful. The additional time spent getting to know the patient lays a foundation for trust, but remember that it's insufficient on its own. Spending time in subsequent visits and making a commitment to patient continuity will ultimately lead to trust equity.

A high level of trust that's established through repeated encounters is not likely to be wiped out with a single negative experience. The patient will be more likely to give the physician the benefit of the doubt when there is substantial trust equity to draw on. The bad experience may lower the equity in the physician's "account." But open communication and continuity with the patient will allow trust to accrue again over time—and a sincere apology will contribute to it.

When patients feel abandoned and cut off from communicating with their doctor, all trust equity is likely to dissipate and the account will be closed. With nothing left to draw on, patients may become resentful and angry, choosing other ways to settle their grievances.

Calculating Trust Equity: Tools for Physicians

Physicians can gauge how well trust equity is accruing in their patient relationships by asking themselves a few questions.

For primary caregivers: Can you put a face with the name of most of your patients without having to refer to the chart for identifying details? If you ran into one of your patients on the street, would you be able to greet him or her by name? When you can't recall a patient's name, can you at least recall something specific or unique about him or her? If you answered no to most of these questions, you might have a problem seeing and hearing authentically. You might question if you take enough time with your patients, or if you simply have too many patients. Or is lack of continuity of care, which prevents you from seeing the same patient in subsequent encounters, to blame?

For physicians in a referral practice (surgeons, gastroenterologists, cardiologists, and so forth): Specialists tend to see a greater number of new patients in any given time period. This doesn't relieve them of the responsibility of establishing and maintaining trust. Continuity, on the other hand, may not be as important for you as it is for primary caregivers. Physicians in referral practice should consider this question: In two years, will this patient remember my name? In other words, are you establishing an effective relationship that will cause a patient to remember you beyond the procedure you performed or the treatment rendered? The answer reflects the degree of connection that you make with your patients. I've seen patients with multiple abdominal scars from various surgeries who could not recall the names of the surgeons. How strange that someone would not remember the name of a person who operated on him or her. What does this say about the relationship?

Recognizing Difficult Physician-Patient Communication

Three clues clearly signal a difficult relationship:

Interruption: Either the doctor or the patient is frequently and/or increasingly interrupting the other.

Repetition: Either party frequently repeats the same statements, often getting louder with each repetition.

Stereotypical responses: Either party (but usually the physician) responds in clichés to disengage the other party (for example, *"Don't worry about that,"* or *"That's just our policy"*).

"Human-Issue-Human" Approach

The "human-issue-human" approach is a useful technique for overcoming problem communications. In a nutshell, you first acknowledge the human, then deal with the issue, and close by focusing on the human again.

For example, when a patient is upset or angry, engage her as a person first and foremost. Call her by her first name if you can. Empathize with her concerns, whether voiced or observed, but reflect her feelings: *"Michelle, I can see that you are very upset."* Verbal validation of the feeling gives the patient an opening to talk to you about her problem. When you demonstrate an understanding of a patient's distress, it helps her feel calmer. When she is authentically engaged, address the problem: *"Michelle, how can I be of assistance in this situation? What do you need from me now?"*

If you are unable to address the issue directly, tell her you will find an answer or engage someone who will be able to help. Taking notes, as long as you pay attention and maintain appropriate eye contact, conveys that you are truly interested and intend to follow up. Tell the patient that you will contact her with your findings.

Finally, refocus on the personal relationship, and close the interaction: *"Michelle, I'm glad you brought this to my attention. I'll do my best. Please don't hesitate to give me additional feedback."*

Conclusive Changes

Of course, I have presented here just a few of the myriad relationship-building tools that should be standard issue with a medical diploma. As health care continues on its inexorable path toward becoming a more patient-centered system, the ability to establish and maintain strong, productive relationships with staff and patients alike will be essential to doctors' professional survival.

In 1998 the Accreditation Council for Graduate Medical

Education adopted "interpersonal/communication" and "professional" skills as core competencies in which graduates must demonstrate proficiency. As medical schools align their curricula with these competencies, new doctors will be emerging from school equipped to handle the "soft" side of medicine in a way that I believe will produce better health care, increased job satisfaction, and lower malpractice costs.

Apology is a fundamental part of the standard repertoire of social communication. I hope someday the phrase *I'm sorry* will be as easy for doctors to say as it is for the rest of the world, because it will signal that we have fully integrated our humanity into our profession.

Reference
1. Pichert J.W., et al.: Understanding the etiology of serious medical events involving children. *Ped Ann* 26:160–172, 1997.

Acknowledgments
(First Edition)

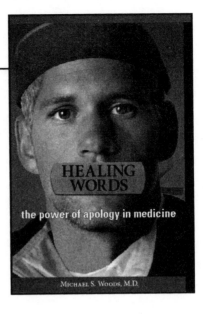

This book wouldn't exist if not for some very important people and their support, both emotionally and financially. Jim Cunningham is a unique individual who sees the value of and believes in my efforts to enhance the health care experience for all stakeholders. There have been many days when, without Jim, I would not have had the energy to continue. His involvement and guidance have suffused me—as well as others—with renewed commitment to our vision. Hilda Brucker, editor, researcher, and teacher, has the patience of Job. I contributed the ideas for this work. Hilda went the extra mile—research, telephone calls, e-mails—all to bolster the original ideas. And then she converted what I gave her into the King's English! What I have learned about writing from Hilda cannot be put into words nor valued in dollars. Bob Viola and Louis Weisberg, both of MVTEN, took what I thought was perfect work and made it "perfecter." Louis worked magic with what he calls "tweaks" that added additional clarity and focus without loss of meaning—and, in fact, perhaps added more meaning. Sarah Dore, a fount of reason and a pragmatist who believes in our mission (and apology!), continually challenges me to think differently. Her grasp of the medical malpractice insurance industry is unparalleled. Her sense of humor is nearly as precious as her advice. And Marcia, Ian, and Jenna who, while listed last, are always first. Marcia, my wife, who supported the family while I chased my dream to make a difference. Who never complained about the need for more investment, whether it was my time, or our money. And the one I still love to be with. Our children remind us daily that there is more to life than money and things. I could live in a refrigerator box with them, as long as I could keep them warm when it was cold, cool when it was hot, and make sure they were never hungry.

In addition to those noted above, others who played a role in this work, in some capacity, include Sue Ann Capizzi; Lisa Chambers Howard; William Gallagher and Dieter Zimmer of Northwest Physician Mutual in Salem, Oregon; and Ray Mazzotta, Darrell Ranum, and Paul Nagle of OHIC in Columbus, Ohio.

Acknowledgments *(Second Edition)*

I would be utterly remiss if I did not first thank all those people who bought the first edition of *Healing Words*. It seems obvious that a second edition would not exist, had it not been for the enthusiastic support of the readers. And I have found that the readers are believers in what *Healing Words* is all about.

The success of the first edition is, in no small way, the result of an incredibly driven and competent young man named David Leander. He mailed thousands of letters, made umpteen telephone calls, and even contacted U.S. senators to make them aware of the book. My thanks to David for his determination and resourcefulness.

Although not involved with the second edition, I remain indebted to Bob Viola and his crew at Polaris Creative (formerly MVTEN). Literally hundreds of readers have commented on the power of the book cover and the message it communicates. More important, I thank them for their unwavering belief in what I attempt to stand for—patient-centered health care.

A special thanks to Donna Hartl, Tony Taglia, Darrin Baim, and Charlie Quinn. And they know why. 'Nuf said.

Cathy Hinckley at Joint Commission Resources called me to see if I would write a book for them on communication, based upon my paper "The DUN Factor." After about five minutes of convincing, she agreed to pitch the second edition of *Healing Words*. And here we are. Thanks to her for her faith and her colleagues at JCR for seeing the value in the book and moving forward so quickly. It is a pleasure to feel like part of a team trying to do the right thing together.

A heartfelt thanks to Alex Valdez, Rick Crabtree, Gary Frank, and Ryan Stevens at St. Vincent Regional Medical Center for allowing me time to write and putting their confidence in me to contribute meaningfully to the organization. Thanks to my partners (Ed Bieniek, Caesar Ursic, Dirk Wassner, Tim Wetherill, and Ray Shapiro) for covering my patients, yet again, while I take time off to spread the word.

Finally, but never last, again . . . or more accurately . . . still Marcia and my children, who put up with countless "Just a minute, Honey's" while I finished yet another sentence. My children who begged to sit on my lap and watch me type—a ruse to simply sit with me (and eventually to beg to watch our digital home movies on the Apple, again). Marcia remains my closest, smartest, best, and nearly flawless advisor, and my children remain my most important teachers. "I'll love you forever, I'll like you for always. As long as I'm living, my babies you'll be."

Resources

Beckman H.B., et al.: The doctor-patient relationship and malpractice. Lessons from plaintiff depositions. *Arch Intern Med* 154:1365–1670, 1994.

Engel B.: *The Power of Apology.* New York: John Wiley & Sons, 2001.

Gallagher T.H., et al.: Patients' and physicians' attitudes regarding the disclosure of medical errors." *JAMA* 289(8):1001–1007, 2003.

Hickson G.B., et al.: Patient complaints and malpractice risk. *JAMA* 287(22):2951–2957, 2002.

Joint Commission Resources: *2006 Comprehensive Accreditation Manual for Hospitals: The Official Handbook.* Oakbrook Terrace, IL: Joint Commission on Accreditation of Healthcare Organizations, 2006.

Jonsen A.R., Siegler M., Winslade W.J.: *Clinical Ethics.* 4th ed. McGraw-Hill Health Professions Division, 1998.

Kraman S.S., Hamm G.: Risk management: Extreme honesty may be the best policy. *Ann Int Med* 131(12):963–967, 1999.

Levinson W., et al.: Physician-patient communication. The relationship with malpractice claims among primary care physicians and surgeons. *JAMA* 277:553–559, Feb. 19, 1997.

Pichert J.W., et al.: Understanding the etiology of serious medical events involving children. *Ped Ann* 26:160–172, 1997.

The SorryWorks! Coalition Web site. http://www.sorryworks. net.

Waitzkin H.: Doctor-patient communication. Clinical implications of social scientific research. *JAMA* 252:2441–2446, 1997.

White M.: Difficult clinician-patient relationships. *Journal of Clinical Outcomes Management* 5(5):32–36, 1998.

Witman A.B., Park D.M., Hardin S.B.: How do patients want physicians to handle mistakes? *Arch Intern Med* 156:2565–2569, 1996.

Zeigler J.: On the run. *The New Physician* pp. 16–21, Mar. 2003.

About the Author

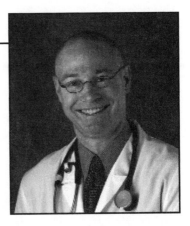

Dr. Michael S. Woods followed his father's footsteps into medicine, earning an M.D. from the University of Kansas. He completed residency training in general surgery at the University of Kansas, followed by a fellowship in hepatobiliary-pancreatic surgery at Virginia Mason Clinic in Seattle. Dr. Woods currently practices surgery at St. Vincent Regional Medical Center in Santa Fe, New Mexico. In addition to his patient care responsibilities, he is the Medical Director of the St. Vincent Surgical Group.

Dr. Woods is a recognized authority on physician personal leadership behavior and communication, patient satisfaction, physician-patient relationships, and novel strategies to reduce medical malpractice. Robert E. Quinn, the M.E. Tracy Collegiate Professor of Organizational Behavior and Human Resource Management at the University of Michigan and author of *Deep Change* and *Change the World*, has noted that Dr. Woods's work in physician leadership "has the power to transform the medical system." Kevin Cashman, the CEO of LeaderSource® and author of *Leadership from the Inside Out*, notes Dr. Woods "provides the inspired vision and practical tools to create a more purposeful, healthy future for us all." His ideas to solve the problems in medical malpractice have been described as "a real breakthrough strategy."

Dr. Woods is the Founder and President of the Center for Physician Leadership (http://www.doctorslead.com), a Santa Fe–based center whose mission is to enable individuals and organizations to navigate to patient-centered excellence by promoting leadership and civility. Dr. Woods has an active speaking career, with clients through the United States. His clients have included the Department of Defense, U.S. Army Medical Command, American Society of Cataract and Refractive Surgery, and the New York Northern Metropolitan Hospital Association.

In addition to *Healing Words*, Dr. Woods is the author of *The DEPO Principle: Applying Personal Leadership Principles to Health Care*, considered an authoritative assessment of the need for physician personal leadership in health care. He is currently revising and updating *The DEPO Principle*. Most recently he co-authored and edited *Cultural Sensitivity: A Guidebook for Physicians & Healthcare Professionals* with Geri-Ann Galanti, Ph.D., a recognized expert in medical anthropology. He has recently completed the development of a comprehensive training program to help organizations achieve Sustained Dynamic Excellence.

In addition to these publications, he has authored numerous articles on leadership development and risk management, and more than 20 peer-reviewed medical papers. He served as a resource for National Public Radio's *This American Life's* segment on apology in health care and has been interviewed by many popular publications, including *Time* and *Self* magazines.

Dr. Woods is a Fellow of the American College of Surgeons and a Member of the International Association of Protocol Consultants.

Dr. Woods may be contacted at mwoods@doctorslead.com or 505/603-8410.

INDEX

A

Abandonment, feelings of, 19, 71, 77–80
Accreditation Council for Graduate Medical Education, 125–126
Airline industry, 101–102
AMA Code of Medical Ethics, 95–97
American College of Physician Executives Patient Trust and
    Safety survey, 59
American Medical Association (AMA) Code of Medical Ethics, 95–97
Anderson, Philip, 47
Anesthesiology error, 89
Anger, 18, 20–21, 24, 48, 59, 61–62, 75–76
Apologies
    as admission of fault, 10, 104
    authentic apologies, 11, 33, 37, 51–52, 65, 86, 102
    barriers and obstacles to, 87–91, 104–105
    benefits of, 35–36, 45, 52
    compelled apologies, 74–75
    components of, 65–76
    culture of civility with, 108–109
    day-to-day use of, 9–10, 40
    delivery of, 72–73
    doctors' use of, 10–11, 50, 126
    disclosure and, 33–37
    history of, 49–50
    litigation reduction with, 11, 35, 39, 52, 57–58, 104–105
    meaning of, 49–50
    motivation for, 62–64
    physicians' use of, 10–11, 50, 126
    programs for, 34–36, 81–86
    rarity of, 49
    resistance to, 39–41, 87–90
    restorative power of, 11, 51–52, 54–56
    situations that call for, 67
    surveys on, 57–59
    timing of, 63, 72–73
    training on how to apologize, 36
    traits that make it difficult to apologize, 41
Apology laws, 87–88, 103–105
Appendectomy malpractice suit, 13–16

ASRS (Aviation Safety Reporting System), 102
Attorneys
    apologies as admission of fault, 10
    public's feelings about, 21
Authentic apologies, 11, 33, 37, 51–52, 65, 86, 102
Authentic body language, 120–121
Authentic communication, 115–121
Authentic listening, 119–120
Authentic writing, 120
Aviation Safety Reporting System (ASRS), 102

B

Banja, John, 90
Body language, authentic, 120–121
Boothman, Richard, 34–37, 84

C

Caring relationships, 17–18, 44–45, 60–61
Cashman, Kevin, 119
Catholic Healthcare West, 89
Cedars-Sinai Medical Center, Los Angeles, 120
Chaos theory, 10
Cholecystectomy, 78–80
Circle of concern®, 21
Circle of control®, 20
Civility
    benefits of, 111–113
    culture of, 107–113
    health outcomes and, 113
    interpretation of, 110–111
    principle of, 110, 113
    transforming health care with, 109–111
Code of Medical Ethics (AMA), 95–97
Communication
    authentic communication, 115–121
    civility, culture of, 107–108
    Code of Medical Ethics (AMA), 95–97
    curriculum for, 125–126
    eye contact, 121
    human-issue-human approach, 124–125
    individual-specific health information, 118
    information needs of patients, 118

informing patients of outcome of care, 97
introduction to patients by physicians, 117
litigation-reduction measures, 82, 84, 85, 86
male vs. female physicians, 64
nonverbal communication, 120–121
physician-to-patient, 12, 18, 77
question-and-answer techniques, 117–118
termination of, 39
transparent communication, 21, 26, 28–30
written communication, 120
Compassion, 48, 60–61
Compelled apologies, 74–75
Compensation, 69–72, 75, 103
Conflict avoidance, 77–78
Consent process, 97–99, 116
Control maintenance by physicians, 117, 118
COPIC Insurance Company, 84–86
Cover-up attempts, 27–28, 55–56, 88
Cultural obstacles to apologies, 87–90
Culture of civility, 107–113

D

DEPO Principle, The (Woods), 40
Disclosure
apologies and, 33–37
barriers and obstacles to, 87–90
benefits of, 35, 93–94
definition, 93
example of, 68
mandatory public disclosure, 100–102
negative connotations of, 93
patient perspective on, 94–95
programs for, 34–36, 81–86, 103
reasons to disclose, 93–94
standards on, 99–100
training on how to disclose, 36
Doctors. *See* physicians
DUN factor, 10

E

Educational remedy, 70–71
Einstein, Albert, 46

Eisenhower, Dwight D., 33
Emotions
component of litigation, 17–19
disengagement by physicians, 45–48
listening, authentic, 119–120
Empathy, 41, 59, 61
Engaged, remaining, 72–74, 77–80
Engel, Beverly, 41, 51, 59, 62, 65, 73
Ethics, 95–97
Eye contact, 121

F

Female physicians, 64
Financial remedy, 71–72
Flexibility, 42
Forni, P. M., 9, 12, 13, 109–110
Functional blindness, 25–26

G

Gallagher, Thomas, 61, 70, 94–95
Gallbladder removal error, 78–80
Guilty conscience, 63

H

Handwriting classes, 120
Health literacy, 44, 116, 118
Health outcomes and relationships, 113
Hickson, Gerald, 19, 56, 77
Honesty dividend, xiv, 84, 89, 103
Humanism, 47–48, 60
Human-issue-human approach, 124–125

I

Ignorance about reason for anger, 75
Indiana University Medical School, 120
Infant death story, 53–54
Informed consent, 97–99, 116
Institute of Medicine (IOM) report, 100–101

INDEX

Insurance
    COPIC Insurance Company, 84–86
    risk management policies, 37
    voided policies for apologies, 10, 11, 96
IOM (Institute of Medicine) report, 100–101

J

Jefferson Medical College, 64
Johns Hopkins Civility Initiative, 109
Joint Commission on Accreditation of Healthcare Organizations, 97

K

Kaiser Hospitals, 89
Kenney, Linda, 89
Kraman, Steve, 34–36

L

Lawsuits. *See* Litigation
Lawyers. *See* Attorneys
Leadership, 42, 44, 109
Leadership from the Inside Out (Cashman), 119
Legal obstacles to apologies, 87–90
Levinson, Wendy, 18
Listening, authentic, 119–120
Litigation
    appendectomy suit, 13–16
    Code of Medical Ethics (AMA), 96–97
    as duels, 50
    effect of apology on, 11, 35, 39, 52, 58–59, 103
    emotional component of, 17–19
    factors in suits, 18–19, 21, 35, 74–75, 77, 112
    fear of, 54–55
    honesty dividend, xiv, 84, 89, 103
    male vs. female physicians, 64
    office visit length and, 18
    patients as drivers of, 20–21
    payment amounts, 82, 83–84, 85–86, 90
    reduction in claims, 11, 35, 39, 52, 58–59, 81–86, 103
    responsibility for, 26
    risk factors, 19

termination of communication, 39
toll on physicians, 50
Wojcieszak suit, 20–25
Lung lesion story, 54–55

M

Male physicians, 64
Malpractice lawsuits. *See* Litigation
Mandatory public disclosure, 100–102
Marcus, Leonard J., 94
Mea Culpa (Tavuchis), 49
Medical errors
   anesthesiology error, 89
   appendectomy malpractice suit, 13–16
   causes of, 57–58, 63, 69, 88
   cholecystectomy error, 78–80
   Code of Medical Ethics (AMA), 95–97
   cover-up attempts, 27–28, 55–56, 88
   deaths from, 100
   debate on how to handle, 24–25
   gallbladder removal error, 78–80
   honesty dividend, xiv, 84, 89, 103
   informing patients of outcome of care, 97
   Jim Wojcieszak, 22–24
   lung lesion story, 54–55
   patient questions about, 94–95
   perfectionism and, 40
   physician as cause of, 57–58, 63, 69
   prevalence of, 17
   prevention of, 95
   toll on physicians, 61, 63
   transparency about, 28–30
Medical Errors and Medical Narcissism (Banja), 90

N

Narcissism, 90
National Practitioner Data Bank, 82
National Practitioner Database Guidebook, 90
Nonverbal communication, 120–121

INDEX

O

Objectivity, 45–46
Office visits, length of, 18, 121

P

Patients
    communication with physicians, 12, 18, 77
    healing process and apologies, 11
    health literacy, 44, 116, 118
    individual-specific health information, 118
    information needs of, 118
    perception of physicians' attitudes, 15, 27, 77–78, 116–117
    perspective on disclosure, 94–95
    relationships with physicians, 17–19, 21, 26, 35, 36, 47–48, 64, 115
Patient Trust and Safety survey (American College of Physician
    Executives), 59
Perfectionism, 40, 41, 43, 90
Personal leadership, 42
Physicians
    apologies, use of, 10–11, 50, 126
    behavior of, 112
    as cause of medical errors, 57–58, 63, 69
    communication with patients, 12, 18, 77
    complaints about, 19
    control maintenance by, 117, 118
    defensive attitude, 14, 90
    handwriting skills of, 120
    ignorance about reason for anger, 75
    introduction to patients, 117
    leadership, 109
    male vs. female, 63–64
    perception of attitudes of, 15, 27, 77–78, 116–117
    qualities of, 40, 42–43
    relationships, quality of, 17–19, 21, 26, 35, 36, 47–48, 64, 115
    toll of litigation on, 50
    toll of medical errors on, 61, 63
    training of, 10, 12, 36, 40, 125–126
    trust equity tools, 123–124
Power of Apology, The (Engel), 51, 59
Professionalism, 41, 43–45
Public disclosure, 100–102

R

Recognition, 65–67
Regret, expression of, 62–63, 67–68
Relationships
    caring relationships, 17–18, 44–45, 59, 60–61
    health outcomes and, 113
    human-issue-human approach, 124–125
    manipulation of, 37
    preserving, 63
    quality of, 17–19, 21, 26, 35, 36, 47–48, 64, 115
    relationship-building tools, 123–125
    research about, 18–19
    trusting relationships, 21, 53–54, 102–103, 121–124
Remain engaged, 71, 72, 77–80
Remedy, 69–72, 75, 103
Respect, 21, 40, 42, 45, 50, 59–60
Responsibility, 60, 68–69
Risk management policies, 34–35, 36–37, 52, 63-64

S

Sincerity, 115
Sorry Works! coalition, 20, 35
Statement of transparency, 69. *See also* Disclosure
Surveys on apologies, 57–59

T

Teamwork, 43
Traits that make it difficult to apologize, 41
Transparency Quotient survey, 30–32
Transparent communication, 21, 26, 28–30
Trust equity tools, 123–124
Trusting relationships, 21, 53–54, 102–103, 121–124

U

University of Michigan Health System, 35, 83–84
University of North Carolina at Chapel Hill, Kenan-Flagler Business
    School, 112

INDEX

V

Vanderbilt University, 59
van Pelt, Frederick, 89
Veterans Affairs Medical Center, Lexington, Kentucky, 35, 81–83, 89

W

Waitzkin, Howard, 117, 118
Win-win solutions, 42
Wojcieszak, Doug, 20–24
Wojcieszak, Jim, 22–24
Writing, authentic, 120

X

XY factor, 63–64

3